Understanding the role of neural activity in the development of the brain has been a major concern of many modern neurobiologists. The reason is plain enough: since the world influences the brain by means of action potentials and synaptic potentials, activity must be the chief cause of the neural changes wrought by experience. In clear and succinct language, Professor Purves explores the hypothesis that neural activity generated by experience modulates the ongoing growth of the brain during maturation, thus sculpting in each of us a unique nervous system according to the events of our early life.

Brain growth is considered at a macroscopic level by examining brain maps and their modular substructure, and at a cellular level by investigating the neuronal interactions that influence the formation and maintenance of these structures. The ways that experience influences the maturation of the brain at both macroscopic and microscopic levels are described, and the conventional wisdom is re-examined. Anyone interested in how the brain stores information will find this book instructive and provocative.

Neural activity and
the growth of the brain

Lezioni Lincee
Sponsored by *Foundazione IBM Italia*
Editor: *Luigi A. Radicati di Brozolo, Scuola Normale Superiore, Pisa*

The Lezioni Lincee arises from lectures given under the auspices of the Accademia Nazionale dei Lincei and is sponsored by *Foundazione IBM Italia*.

The lectures, given by international authorities, will range on scientific topics from mathematics and physics through to biology and economics. The books are intended for a broad audience of graduate students and faculty members, and are meant to provide a '*mise au point*' for the subjects they deal with.

The symbol of the Accademia, the lynx, is noted for its sharp-sightedness; the volumes in the series will be penetrating studies of scientific topics of contemporary interest.

Already published

Chaotic Evolution and Strange Attractors: D. Ruelle
Introduction to Polymer Dynamics: P. de Gennes
The Geometry and Physics of Knots: M. Atiyah
Attractors for Semigroups and Evolution Equations:
    O. Ladyzhenskaya
Asymptotic Behaviour of Solutions of Evolutionary Equations:
    M.I. Vishik
Half a Century of Free Radical Chemistry: D.H.R. Barton in
    collaboration with S.I. Parekh
Bound Carbohydrate in Nature: L. Warren

Neural activity and the growth of the brain

DALE PURVES

Department of Neurobiology,
Duke University Medical Center,
Durham, North Carolina, USA

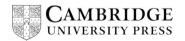
CAMBRIDGE
UNIVERSITY PRESS

Published by the Press Syndicate of the University of Cambridge
The Pitt Building, Trumpington Street, Cambridge CB2 1RP
40 West 20th Street, New York, NY 10011-4211, USA
10 Stamford Road, Oakleigh, Melbourne 3166, Australia

First published 1994

Printed in Great Britain at the University Press, Cambridge

A catalogue record for this book is available from the British Library

Library of Congress cataloguing in publication data

Purves, Dale.
Neural activity and the growth of the brain / Dale Purves.
    p.   cm. – (Lezioni Lincee)
Includes bibliographical references and index.
ISBN 0 521 45496 4 (hardback). – ISBN 0 521 45570 7 (pbk.)
1. Brain – Growth.   2. Neuroplasticity.   3. Neural circuitry.
I. Title.   II. Series.
[DNLM: 1. Brain – physiology.   2. Mental processes – physiology.
WL 300 P9857n   1944]
QP356.25 P87   1994
612.8'2 – dc20
DNLM/DLC for Library of Congress   93-34582 CIP

ISBN 0 521 45496 4   hardback
ISBN 0 521 45570 7   paperback

Contents

viii   *Contents*

Preface

These lectures, sponsored by the Accademia Nazionale dei Lincee and IBM, Italia, were delivered in June 1992 at the Scoula Normale Superiore in Pisa, Italy. Their purpose was to consider the relationship between the postnatal growth of the nervous system, particularly the brain, and the remarkable ability of this organ to store large amounts of information as animals mature. The hypothesis examined is that experience-related neural activity modulates the growth of neuropil in the brain, most probably by its influence on trophic relationships between nerve cells. In this view, the end result of such activity-dependent growth is the orchestrated creation of additional circuitry during maturation, which permanently encodes the effects of early experience.

I am particularly grateful for the opportunity of spending the week of the lectures at the Instituto di Neurofisiologia del CNR, which is under the direction of Lamberto Maffei. My interactions with so many fine faculty members and bright students were especially useful and rewarding. I should also like to thank my colleagues in the laboratory for many valuable suggestions during the preparation of these talks.

Dale Purves
Durham, North Carolina

Introduction

Whatever information our brains possess is stored in the almost unimaginably complex circuitry of this unique organ. A corollary of this truism is that the storage of information derived from an animal's experience in the world must be initiated by the effects of the neural activity on brain circuitry.

There are, in principle, two ways that neural activity could influence neural connectivity: functional modification of existing circuitry and/or the elaboration of novel circuitry. That the mammalian brain might avail itself of both these strategies for storing information makes sense in terms of the needs of an animal, which must permanently retain some of what happens to it during life, and yet must learn, remember, and forget on a much briefer time-scale (seconds, minutes or days). Modification of existing circuits (a circuit is defined here as a set of neural connections serving some common purpose) might be expected when the desired neural change must be rapidly effected and readily reversed. Novel circuitry would presumably take longer to create and be more difficult to expunge. Moreover, the elaboration of novel circuitry to store information might be more likely to characterize an animal's early life, when the brain is growing rapidly and life-long propensities are being molded by individual circumstances. It is during this period that an individual 'personality' emerges, setting up patterns of behavior that tend to endure. The relative permanence of such information is apparent not only as memory, but in the recalcitrance of the fully formed human personality to change; witness the difficulty of behavioral reformation by psychotherapy and other attempts to re-educate adults in some fundamental way. The neural changes wrought by early experience to a considerable extent determine who we are.

These lectures explore the second of these developmental strategies, namely the relationship of neural activity to the elaboration of neural circuitry. The hypothesis put forward is that the neural activity modulates the growth of nerve cells and neural circuits, ultimately affecting the overall growth of the brain and its constituent parts. By modulating neuronal growth, the activity associated with experience permanently alters the circuitry of the developing brain, thereby storing information.

Circumstantial evidence supporting this view has come from several areas of modern neurobiology. First, destroying afferent inputs during the development of sensory systems generally causes atrophy of the target regions of the brain (reviewed in Purves and Lichtman, 1985a, Chapter 8). Second, electrical activity can influence the growth of neurons and their targets under experimental conditions (reviewed in Purves, 1988, Chapter 8). Third, activity modulates the growth of other excitable cells such as smooth, cardiac and skeletal muscle fibers, which hypertrophy or atrophy according to their level of stimulation (Close, 1972; Goldberg *et al.*, 1975; Burke, 1983; Jones *et al.*, 1989). And finally, deprivation of normal experience in early life can change some aspects of neural circuitry and behavior in a variety of animals (reviewed in Sherman and Spear, 1983; Purves and Lichtman, 1985a, Chapter 14).

Despite these tantalizing observations, the influence of activity on brain growth and information storage (as contrasted with its influence on competition and selection) has never been thoroughly examined. This is not to say that other investigators have not considered the possibility that experience might influence the growth of the brain and its constituent parts. In the late 1940s, the psychologist Donald Hebb and his students proposed that experience could affect the structure of the brain (Hebb, 1949; see also Juraska, 1987; Tees, 1990). The view (and the experimental paradigm) advanced by this school of psychology, which has subsequently attracted many adherents, is that an 'enriched' environment embellishes neural circuitry, whereas an 'impoverished' environment fails to do so. For reasons that are as much sociological as scientific, this general perspective has not been embraced by most neurobiologists: the large body of work on the effects of enriched environments on the brain is infrequently referred to in the mainstream neurobiological literature, although it has received its fair share of attention from psychologists. More generally, the idea that variations in the size of the brain and its parts might be related to the talents of especially accomplished individuals has a long and fascinating history (Gould, 1977). The experiments I am going to describe were not motivated by the nominal effects of 'enriched' environments or the possible relation of brain size and accomplishment; nonetheless, these investigations represent other, earlier approaches to the same general issue.

The overall aim of these four lectures, then, is to examine the idea that the growth of the brain is normally influenced by experience-dependent neural activity in early life. If activity modulates the growth of neurons and their connections in a continuously graded manner, then a mechanism – the activity-dependent growth of neural circuitry – will have been established to explain how experience leads to the permanent storage of information in the developing nervous system.

Lecture I

Maps

I have divided these talks into four parts concerned with brain maps, modules, trophic interactions and neural activity, respectively. This sequence begins with a consideration of growth at a generally macroscopic level – i.e., of brain maps and their modular substructure. The argument then turns to the cellular interactions that influence the formation of maps and modules, and finally to the role of activity (and experience) in this process.

Brain growth and its potential significance

Brain growth is a concept that all of you are familiar with. When we think of brain growth, however, most neurobiologists probably do so in the context of prenatal development. Indeed, the growth of the brain is quite phenomenal during embryonic life (Figure 1.1; Cowan, 1979). Less noticed has been the extent of postnatal brain growth. Figure 1.2A shows the human brain at birth and in a child of 6, redrawn from J. LeRoy Conel's monographs on human brain development (Conel, 1939–1967). This picture shows at a glance the magnitude of brain growth during the first few years of life. The neonatal human brain weighs about 350 grams on average; in adult males the brain typically weighs 1400 grams (the average values are slightly lower for females, at least in part because of average differences in body size) (Krogman, 1941; Pakkenberg and Voight, 1964; Dekaban and Sadowsky, 1978). Extensive postnatal brain growth is not limited to humans; the average weight of the brain of a mouse also increases by a

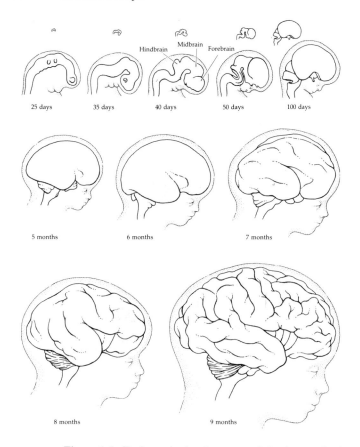

Figure 1.1. Embryonic development of the human brain. The diagrams in this sequence are about four-fifths life-size; the lower diagrams in the first row are enlarged for clarity. Assuming that the fully developed human brain contains approximately 100 billion neurons and that these do not divide after birth, the developing brain must add an average of 250 000 neurons per minute of early development. Much of embryonic brain growth, therefore, reflects this remarkable proliferation of nerve cells. In primates, however, the generation of nerve cells in the cerebral cortex ceases well before birth. Any subsequent growth must therefore be attributed to other processes. (After Cowan, 1979.)

factor of about four during postnatal maturation (Pomeroy *et al.*, 1990).

Not only is postnatal brain growth remarkable by the simple measure of weight, it is also long lasting. Figure 1.2B represents a heroic effort in the 1970s to gather normative values of human brain size throughout life (Dekaban and Sadowsky, 1978). These authors collected information about the brains of some 5000 patients who came to autopsy over a 10-year period in the Washington, DC area. After eliminating cases that might have been neurologically abnormal, they were left with about 2600 brains, from which they made this graph, plotting brain weight as a function of age. Although our brains grow most rapidly during the first few years of life, growth (measured here by weight) continues to an appreciable degree for the better part of two decades.

On what processes is the postnatal growth of the brain based, and why should ongoing brain growth be an important concern of developmental neurobiologists? First, one can say with assurance that the postnatal growth of the brain does not depend upon the proliferation of additional neurons. Primates, at least, are born with most or all the nerve cells that they are ever going to have. Studies using tritiated thymidine autoradiography to determine cellular 'birthdates' have shown that by the end of gestation in the monkey (and presumably in humans), all the neurons of the cerebral cortex and most other brain regions have been generated (Rakic, 1974, 1985).

If postnatal growth does not involve the generation of additional nerve cells, what then does it signify? The answer is a number of different things – among them the ongoing generation of glial cells, the myelination of axons, and the addition of more vasculature and connective tissue. Each of these processes no doubt contributes to the increasing postnatal size of the brain. But from the point of view of developmental neurobiology, surely the most interesting aspect of

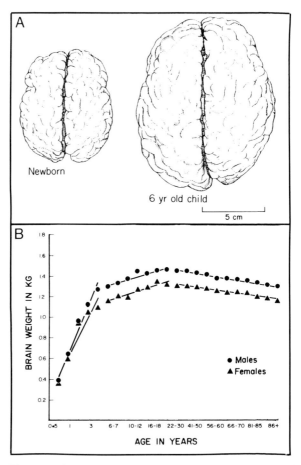

Figure 1.2. Postnatal growth of the human brain. (A) Dorsal view of a normal brain at birth (left) and at age 6 years (right). (B) The duration of human brain growth (according to brain weight). The growth of the brain (here based on 2603 neurologically normal subjects) continues for a decade or more.

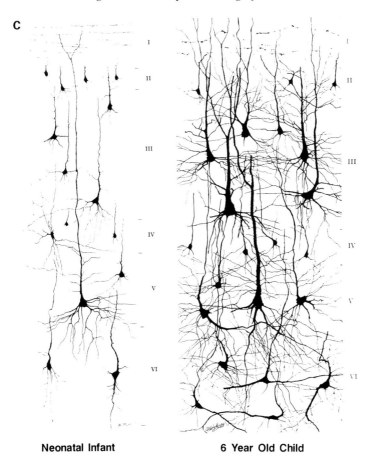

Neonatal Infant   **6 Year Old Child**

Figure 1.2. (*cont.*) (C) Tracings of Golgi-stained neurons in the parietal cortex of a neonatal human brain (left) and the brain of a 6-year old (right). The marked enlargement of neurons and their branches during maturation implies that much postnatal brain growth arises from the ongoing elaboration of neuropil. (A and C are after Conel, 1939–1967; B after Dekaban and Sadowsky, 1978.)

postnatal brain growth is that the *neurons themselves are growing* (Figure 1.2C). More particularly, the *neuropil* is growing, presumably reflecting the establishment of more and more circuitry as the animal matures. ('Neuropil' is a useful term that refers to the dense matrix of axons, dendrites and synapses that lies between the nerve cell bodies in the brain and other neural tissues.)

The point I wish to emphasize, and it is a theme I shall return to repeatedly in these lectures, is the potential significance of this ongoing creation of novel circuitry. We each accumulate a tremendous amount of information as we grow to maturity; I will argue that the modulation of neuronal growth by neural activity is how much of this information storage comes about.

A contrary view of brain development

Every good argument needs a foil, and it may be useful to bring up at the outset what I take to be the opposing (and conventional) position in this particular inquiry. Without wishing to ascribe the conventional view to any particular people (I have certainly endorsed aspects of it over the years), a great many neurobiologists (and others) imagine the basic strategy of neural development to be a *selective* one. The biological strategy generally envisioned is that the brains of humans and other mammals comprise a large initial *excess* of synaptic connections and circuits. Then, during development, those connections that are particularly useful to an animal are selected and sustained, whereas the others are removed. This process has been compared to natural selection, and is widely referred to as 'neural Darwinism'. The Darwinian view has been elaborated in numerous papers in the primary literature, in reviews and in several books, and in the popular press (see, for example, Young 1973, 1979; Changeux *et al.*, 1973; Changeux and Danchin, 1976; Edelman, 1978; Edelman, 1987;

Changeux, 1985; Gazzaniga, 1993). Although I will argue that the importance of the selection of useful circuitry from an initial excess is much exaggerated, pouring cold water on neural Darwinism is certainly not my main concern. Quite the contrary; my goal is to present evidence for the *constructive* role of activity in brain growth, and to point out the merits of the constructionist perspective. Nonetheless, it may add some interest to recognize that there is an opposing position to what I have to say, that this view is presently quite popular, and that it appears to be wrong.

Brain maps

With that general introduction to brain growth, the major topic I want to discuss here is the organization of the brain into maps, and the growth of the brain in relation to this underlying topography. Since the late 19th century, neurologists have recognized that specific neural functions are localized in the brain, and that in many such regions there is a further topographic arrangement of functional areas such that the body and its parts are systematically represented.

Figure 1.3A shows two maps in humans that have been particularly important in both clinical practice and basic research, the primary motor and somatic sensory maps that span the central sulcus on the dorsolateral surface of each hemisphere. As techniques in this century have allowed increasingly accurate delineation of such sensory and motor areas, people naturally asked how much cortical space within the map is allotted to the function of a particular body part such as the hand, the arm, the face, or the trunk. Work earlier in this century showed that the allocation of cortical space is not strictly proportional to the geometry of the body, but that it is more closely related to the importance of that body part for the animal (which is, in turn, related to the amount of peripheral sensory and motor machinery involved – e.g.,

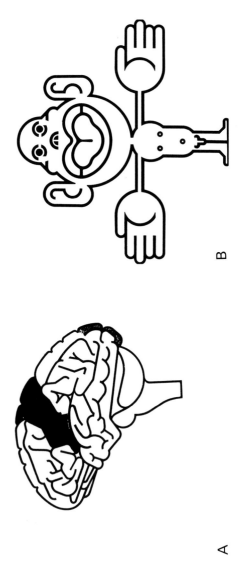

A

B

Figure 1.3. The primary motor and sensory cortex in the human brain. (A) These areas (stipple for sensory and grey for motor) indicate the location and amount of cortex devoted to the initial processing of information related to the sensory structures and muscles that monitor and motivate the body. (B) The homunculus of the human somatic sensory–motor cortex. Mapping studies carried out in patients undergoing surgery have shown that the amount of cortical space devoted to different functions within the primary sensory and motor cortex is proportional to the importance of that function in species-specific behavior. (After Corsi, 1991.)

muscle fibers, sensory receptors, peripheral axons and so on) (Woolsey, 1958). The cortical representation of the hand, for example, which is especially important for us because of the manipulations we must do to succeed in life, is relatively large compared to the representation of the proximal limbs. Similarly, relatively more cortical space is allocated to the sensory-motor apparatus of speech and facial expression than to the sensory-motor apparatus of the trunk. Such facts are usually represented graphically in a cartoon of the so-called 'homunculus' (meaning little man) (Figure 1.3B). The figurine reflects the apportionment of cortical space for either the primary somatic sensory or motor cortex, and is based on the work of neurosurgeons who carefully mapped the cortex in humans with electrophysiological techniques (e.g., Penfield and Boldrey, 1937).

The existence of maps, and the disproportionate representation of various sensory-motor (and presumably other) functions within maps, raises three interesting questions about the nature of brain growth. First, is the growth of maps during development simply in proportion to their initial dimensions, or do some regions grow more than others? In particular, do the regions that are 'over-represented' in maturity, i.e., that have particular significance for the animal, grow more than those that are less important? Second, if, as turns out to be the case, such regions *do* grow more than the rest of the brain, why might this be? Finally, and please note the speculative nature of this last question, might differential growth be related to the storage of information in the maturing brain?

Measurement of maps in the developing brain

The human brain is perhaps the least favorable material in which to explore these questions, not only because human brains are relatively difficult to obtain, but because the geometrical complexity of our highly convoluted cerebral cortex

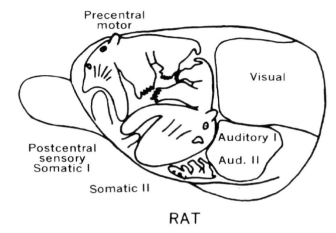

RAT

Figure 1.4. The brains of other mammals, like the human brain, comprise a number of maps. Some of the major cortical maps in the rodent are indicated in this lateral view of the rat brain. Most important for present purposes are the primary motor and sensory maps. (cf. Figure 1.3). (After Woolsey, 1958.)

makes the precise measurement of maps quite difficult. Despite its neat appearance in textbooks, the homunculus shown in Figure 1.3 is a composite of approximate information acquired in conscious patients at the operating table undergoing surgery for epilepsy or some other condition under local anesthesia. Although non-invasive imaging methods are now changing the situation, a precise delineation of somatotopic maps in humans is simply not feasible at present.

One can, however, make quite precise cortical maps in experimental animals, most especially in rodents. Figure 1.4 is a diagram of the rat brain in the same orientation as the human brain in Figure 1.3A. The maps that are apparent in humans exist in other mammals, in roughly the same locations. My colleagues and I chose to study the rat for two reasons. First, because it is readily available for laboratory work, and

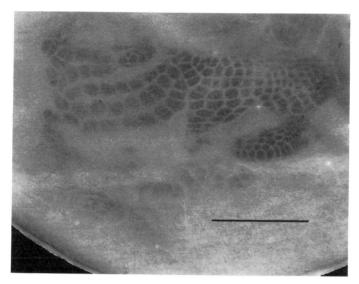

Figure 1.5. The primary somatic sensory map in the rat. Tangential section through layer IV of the rat cortex, stained by SDH histochemistry. This low-power view shows the map in relation to the flattened hemisphere as a whole (anterior is to the right; ventral is up). Scale bar = 2 mm.

second, because the primary somatic sensory map in the rat brain – unlike that in the brains of humans and other primates – can actually be *seen* (Figure 1.5). This primary somatic sensory map (or S1) is the first cortical station for processing information derived (for the most part) from the body's mechanosensory receptors (i.e., sensory endings that respond to mechanical forces such as touch, pressure, stretch and vibration).

The rat brain shown in Figure 1.5 has been flattened into a pancake, sectioned in the plane of the pancake, and stained for succinic dehydrogenase reactivity (a mitochondrial enzyme that figures importantly in Lecture IV). Following such staining, one can see within the brain a representation of the animal's entire body; the 'ratunculus', if you like (Welker, 1971; Wallace, 1987; Dawson and Killackey, 1987). The cortical representation of the head of the animal, the lower jaw, the forepaw, the trunk, and the hindpaw can all be seen clearly, thanks to darkly staining elements within the map called barrels (Woolsey and Van der Loos, 1970). I will have a good deal more to say about barrels later, but for the moment it is sufficient to recognize that their prominence in the rodent brain allows one to visualize the somatic sensory map by virtue of a simple histochemical procedure. Because the representation of the entire body is revealed by such staining, the somatic sensory map and its elements can be measured with considerable accuracy.

To examine how such maps grow, my colleagues and I took a large number of juvenile (1-week-old) rats and compared the somatic sensory map with the map in fully mature (10–12-week-old) animals (Riddle *et al.*, 1992). The general question we sought to answer is whether the map grows uniformly, like the surface of a balloon that is being inflated, or whether some parts of the map grow more than others. Figure 1.6 shows a representative juvenile cortex and a representative adult; clearly, the primary somatic sensory (S1) map grows substantially over this period in postnatal life, increasing in size by a factor of nearly two. It is not obvious from this picture, however, whether all parts of the map grow equally: the geometry is sufficiently complex so that the answer is difficult to discern by simple inspection. We therefore digitized the map so that an image analysis system could measure precisely the areas of cortex devoted to different functions by counting the number of pixels in each of the more obvious representations within the map.

The first issue we considered is whether the S1 map as a whole grows to the same degree as the rest of the neocortex, the most recently evolved part of the cerebral cortex in

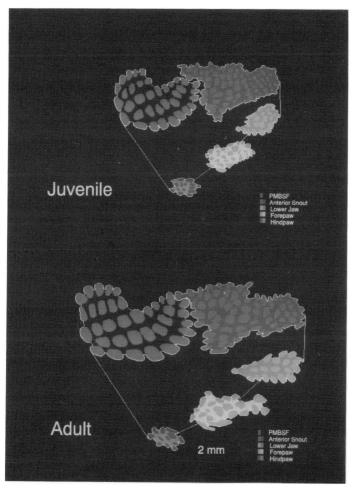

Figure 1.6. The primary somatic sensory map in representative juvenile and adult rats showing overall change in the
size of the map during postnatal maturation. *Top* Juvenile
map (1-week-old animal). *Bottom* Adult map (11-week-old
animal). Whereas the overall growth of S1 is apparent, the
differential growth of its component parts is not; these
differences can be brought out only by detailed measurement. (From Riddle *et al.*, 1992.)

mammals and its major component. We could answer this question by measuring the area of S1 in juvenile and adult animals, and comparing its growth to that of the rest of the neocortex (measured by cutting serial sections through the entire brain, and calculating the full cortical surface area). We found a significant difference between the growth of S1 and the remainder of the cortical mantle: the average area of S1 increased from about 12.5 mm^2 to 22.8 mm^2 (an 83% increment), whereas the entire neocortex of each hemisphere increased from 108 mm^2 to 187 mm^2 (a 73% increment).

The second issue we examined is whether the several major somatic representations evident in S1 (the whiskerpad, anterior snout, lower jaw, forepaw and hindpaw representations – see Figures 1.6 and 1.7) all grow to the same extent. Our interest in this question concerned the ultimate size of each representation. Just as more space in our brains is allotted to the sensory-motor apparatus of speech, facial expression and manipulation, so the configuration of the 'ratunculus' indicates those body parts that are particularly important to a rat. The representation of the whiskerpad, for example, occupies much more cortical space than the representation of the hindpaw (although the whiskerpad is actually smaller than the plantar surface of the hindpaw in a full-grown rat). Measurements of the percent increase in the area of these different regions during maturation show that they do not all grow to the same degree. The whiskers of the animal's snout are the most obviously 'over-represented' peripheral structures in the rat brain, and it is these regions in the somatic sensory map that grow most in the course of maturation (Table 1.1). The hand is over-represented in the homunculus, presumably because we humans depend so heavily on manipulating things. The rat, however, is a nocturnal animal that typically traverses narrow spaces in the dark, but does little manipulation. The rat, therefore, depends on mechanosensory information from its whiskers for survival (Vincent, 1912), and a lot of cortical space is devoted to processing this information.

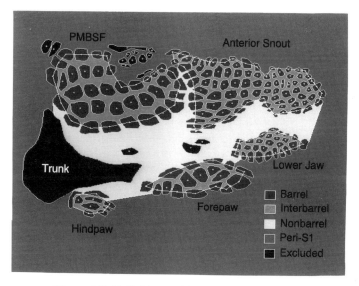

Figure 1.7. Definitions of the rat primary somatic sensory cortex allowing detailed measurements of its component parts. Sections such as the one shown in Figure 1.5 are traced and the complete map digitized and color coded for analysis. For present purposes, S1 as a whole is defined by: (1) the lateral boundary of the head representation; (2) a line between the most posterior medial barrel in the whiskerpad representation (PMBSF) and the most posterior barrel in the hindpaw representation; (3) the medial boundary of the paw representations and a line between the centroids of the hindpaw and forepaw regions; (4) a line between the centroids of the forepaw and lower jaw representations; and (5) the anterior boundary of the lower jaw representation and a line between the most anterior barrel in the lower jaw representation and the most anterior barrel in the head representation. The overall area of S1 is measured by filling in this outline. The area of the nonbarrel cortex within S1 is defined as the area of S1 minus the sum of the areas of the major somatic representations. (From Riddle *et al.*, 1993.)

Table 1.1. *Differences in the average areal growth of each of the major somatic representations in the primary somatic sensory cortex of the rat. (The data presented in Tables 1.1– 1.3 are based on the analysis of 55 hemispheres from juvenile rats and 57 from adult animals. Standard errors of the mean are given.) (From Riddle* et al., *1992.)*

| Representation | Area of each representation (mm^2) | | % Increase |
	Juvenile	Adult	
Whiskerpad	3.04 ± 0.07	5.60 ± 0.10	84
Anterior snout	2.27 ± 0.05	4.36 ± 0.10	92
Lower jaw	0.73 ± 0.02	1.38 ± 0.03	89
Forepaw	0.92 ± 0.03	1.51 ± 0.04	64
Hindpaw	0.24 ± 0.01	0.41 ± 0.02	71

The third issue we examined is whether the modular elements (barrels) within the representations grow to the same extent as the surrounding, 'background' cortex. I did not say much about barrels earlier, and this is perhaps a good time to elaborate on what they signify. Each one of these elements that stains so intensely for the succinic dehydrogenase (SDH) reaction product (see Figure 1.5) is related to a special sensor in the periphery, most often a whisker hair (Woolsey and Van der Loos, 1970). Barrels, however, are not 'hair specific'; the barrel-like structures in the paw representations, for instance, probably represent individual digital pads (Dawson and Killackey, 1987). Nor are barrels simply cortical regions that stain heavily for an enzyme reaction product. Each barrel (there are about 200 in the rat S1) is an intrinsic structure within layer IV of the cortex that can be seen in a variety of ways. Most barrels in the rat parietal cortex appear as a region in which the cell bodies have been partially excluded from a central core that is largely neuropil (although see Megirian *et al.*, 1977) (Figure 1.8). Thus these regions represent cortical

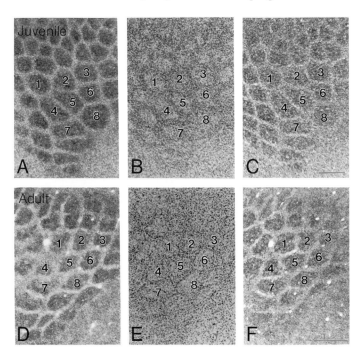

Figure 1.8. Enzymatic and cytoarchitectonic appearance of cortical barrels in both juvenile (1-week-old) animals (A–C) and adult (10–12-week-old) animals (D–F). (A and D): sections of flattened cortex stained for succinic dehydrogenase activity; barrels shown are in the representation of the anterior snout. (B) and (E): cytoarchitectonic definition of barrels in subjacent sections revealed by Nissl staining. (C) and (F): sections adjacent to the ones shown in B and E, stained for cytochrome oxidase activity. Numbers indicate corresponding barrels in each of the three serial sections from the juvenile and adult cortices. Such methods show that barrels are structurally and metabolically distinct elements within the S1 map. Scale bars: A–C, 250 μm; D–F 500 μm. (From Riddle *et al.*, 1992.)

Table 1.2. *Differences in average barrel and interbarrel areal growth in the primary somatic sensory cortex of the rat. (From Riddle* et al., *1992.)*

	Sum of area (mm^2)		
	Juvenile	Adult	% Increase
Barrels	4.74 ± 0.11	9.16 ± 0.15	93
Interbarrels	2.48 ± 0.07	4.10 ± 0.9	65

areas enriched in neuropil devoted to those sensors that are especially useful to the rat, given its mode of existence.

Barrels, like the somatic sensory cortex as a whole, also grow during maturation (Figure 1.9). We could therefore ask whether they increase in area to the same extent as the surrounding cortex. Table 1.2 shows that the cortical representations of these special sensors grow much more than the surrounding (interbarrel) cortex, and indeed more than any other region of S1. We could also ask whether the barrels in different S1 representations grow to different degrees. In fact, the barrels in the head representations grow substantially more during maturation than the barrels in the paw regions (Table 1.3), in accord with the fact that the head representation grows to a greater degree than the other regions of S1 (see Table 1.1).

Four points can be drawn from these observations on the postnatal growth of the rat primary somatic sensory cortex. First, to a small, but significant degree, S1 grows more than the rest of the neocortex. Second, some S1 representations grow more than others, the head representations growing more than the paw representations. Third, the cortical representations of special sensors (barrels) grow more than the

Table 1.3. *Differential barrel growth in the major somatic representations in the primary somatic sensory cortex of the rat. (From Riddle et al., 1992.)*

| Representation | Average barrel area (mm^2) | | % Increase |
	Juvenile	Adult	
Whiskerpad	0.057 ± 0.001	0.112 ± 0.002	96
Anterior snout	0.017 ± 0.001	0.036 ± 0.001	112
Lower jaw	0.016 ± 0.001	0.032 ± 0.001	100
Forepaw	0.024 ± 0.001	0.038 ± 0.001	58
Hindpaw	0.014 ± 0.001	0.021 ± 0.001	50

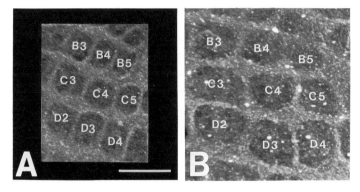

Figure 1.9. The growth of the identified barrels between 1 and 10–12 postnatal weeks. (A) Specific barrels in the whiskerpad representation (barrels B3–B5, C3–C5, D2–D4) in a representative juvenile (1-week-old) animal. (B) The same set of barrels in a representative adult (11-week-old) animal. Note the marked enlargement in barrel cross-sectional area during postnatal maturation. Scale bar = 0.5 mm. (From Riddle *et al.*, 1992.)

surrounding cortex. And finally, barrels grow more in the representations that grow most overall. These several findings all support the view that cortical regions that are particularly important to an animal (and are, therefore, most 'used') grow most during maturation.

Conclusion

To come back to the three questions that I posed at the outset, this evidence in the rat provides an answer to the issue of whether postnatal cortical growth is simply a proportional increase: some cortical regions clearly grow more than others as the animal matures. The second question was *why* some regions of the brain might grow preferentially. I have suggested that the answer may lie in the relative importance of the representation in question to the animal, the most 'significant' (and, therefore, most practiced) regions growing the most. The final question I asked is whether differential brain growth might be related to information storage. If the greater growth of some regions of cortical maps arises (at least in part) because they are more heavily used, then the differential growth of maps may indicate, in a rudimentary sense, how the lessons of experience are encoded in the brain.

I should perhaps emphasize that differential growth must, from a more general point of view, be only a minor factor in the overall development of the brain. In the main, the brain develops in size – and every other respect – according to a diverse set of developmental mechanisms that operates in the same way on all members of a species. These intrinsic mechanisms must, by any calculation, be the major determinant of brain form and function. Indeed, studies of identical twins have provided strong quantitative support for the predominence of nature over nurture in our own development (see, for example, Dunn and Plomin, 1990). On the other hand, the neurological differences in the brain endengered by experience, however small their contribution to the determination of phenotype, are nonetheless of overwhelming importance for us as human beings. Appreciating these differences may well depend on evaluating and understanding very small differential effects on brain growth.

Lecture II

Modules

In this second lecture, I want to turn from maps to consider in more detail the modular substructure that characterizes many somatotopically arranged cortical regions. I will indicate in a moment why it is important to look at brain growth from this perspective. Let me begin, however, with a more general consideration of modules, their discovery and the interpretation of these strikingly patterned arrangements.

Discovery and definition

An iterated arrangement of some brain regions was noticed a long time ago, first in the olfactory bulb by C. Golgi (1874), and some decades later by the Spanish neuroanatomist R. Lorente de Nó, who emphasized iterated vertical patterns in his monograph on the rat cortex (Lorente de Nó, 1922; see also 1949). The modern discovery of the modular arrangement of cortex, however, is generally attributed to V. Mountcastle (1957). In studies of the cat and monkey somatic sensory cortex in the 1950s, Mountcastle found that when he penetrated the cortex with a microelectrode held perpendicular to the surface, all the cells that he recorded along a vertical track tended to have the same qualities. They shared the same receptive field, responded to the same modality of cutaneous stimulation, and had similar response latencies. When he moved his electrode to another spot, the properties of the nerve cells were usually different, but they again shared these common characteristics. At each point, then, there was a vertical organization of cells with similar properties; Mount-castle called this arrangement 'columnar'.

Shortly thereafter, D. Hubel and T. Wiesel, in their studies of the visual system (1962, 1963), confirmed Mountcastle's view that the cortex is organized in a columnar fashion (see also Hubel *et al.*, 1977; LeVay *et al.*, 1978; Hubel, 1988). As in Mountcastle's work, microelectrodes penetrating along a vertical track recorded from cells that tended to respond in the same manner, in this case to a particular orientation of the stimulus in the visual field. When the electrode was moved to another site, they again found neurons that responded maximally to a particular stimulus, but now in a different orientation. Tangential penetrations of the cortex encountered cells with gradually changing orientation preferences, as if the electrode were traversing a series of orientation columns. Soon after these observations, Hubel and Wiesel described an iterated arrangement, the ocular dominance columns, which has since become the most thoroughly studied columnar cortical architecture (op. cit). Then, in the early 1980s, Hubel, J. Horton and others (M. Wong-Riley was really the first to notice this aspect of cortical organization; see Livingstone and Hubel, 1984) discovered another class of iterated unit in the visual cortex that they called 'blobs' (Horton, 1984; Hendrickson, 1985).

Subsequently, a wide variety of such repeating patterns has been described, several examples of which are shown in Figure 2.1. Panel A shows ocular dominance columns in the rhesus monkey visual cortex, made apparent by the transport of tritiated proline injected into one eye (the light stripes are related to the injected eye, and the dark stripes to the uninjected eye) (LeVay *et al.*, 1978). The distance from one ocular dominance column to the next is on the order of 300 μm in the monkey (the other panels are all at the same magnification). Panel B shows blobs in the visual cortex of the squirrel monkey, made visible by cytochrome oxidase histochemistry.

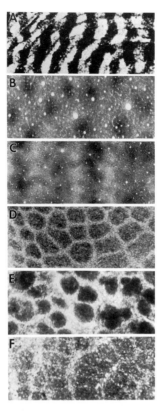

Figure 2.1. Examples of modular circuitry in the mammalian brain. (A) Ocular dominance columns in layer IV in the primary visual cortex (V1) of a rhesus monkey (autoradiography after injection of radioactive proline into one eye). (B) Blobs in layers II–III in the primary visual cortex of a squirrel monkey (cytochrome oxidase histochemistry). (C) Stripes in layers II–III in the secondary visual cortex (V2) of a squirrel monkey (cytochrome oxidase histochemistry). (D) Barrels in layer IV in the primary sensory cortex of a rat (succinic dehydrogenase histochemistry). (E) Glomeruli in the olfactory bulb of a mouse (Sudan Black staining). (F) Barreloids in the ventrobasal nucleus in the thalamus of a rat (succinic dehydrogenase histochemistry). (From Purves *et al.*, 1992.)

Again, the dimensions of these modules are several hundred microns. Panel C shows the thick and thin stripes in the secondary visual cortex of the squirrel monkey, and panel D shows (for comparison) the barrels in the rodent brain that I discussed in the last lecture. Barrels incidentally, are found not just in the rat, but in a variety of other mammals (Woolsey *et al.*, 1975). Panel E shows the modular circuitry in another laminated telencephalic structure, the olfactory bulb. These elements are called glomeruli, and I will say more about them a little later on in this lecture. Finally, panel F is a section through a subcortical structure, the thalamus, showing the so-called barreloids. Barreloids are iterated thalamic modules in this major relay from periphery to cortex that project to the corresponding cortical barrels (see Panel D).

Table 2.1 gives a fuller indication of the variety of modular circuitry that has now been described in the brain. In addition to the somatosensory columns, barrels, orientation columns, ocular dominance stripes, blobs and stripes already mentioned, similar patterns have been found in the auditory, entorhinal, frontal, and parietal cortex; other subcortical units occur in the caudate/putamen and superior colliculus. Although the list in Table 2.1 is not inclusive (more and more examples of these elements are being described as new techniques are applied to previously unexamined regions of the brain), it conveys the point that modular arrangements of circuitry, particularly cortical circuitry, are widespread indeed.

The significance of modularity

What do these arrangements signify? Here, I think, one has to be frank and admit that, despite 30 years of intense investigation and a great deal of speculation, no one really knows (see Purves *et al.*, 1992). The grand purposes imagined for modularity in various regions of cortex notwithstanding (a

Table 2.1. *Some examples of iterated circuitry in the mammalian brain*

Modular type	Location	Physiologically identified	Anatomically identified	Orders in which found	References
Cortical					
Somatosensory columns	S1	Yes	No	Carnivores, rodents, primates	Mountcastle, 1957
Barrels	S1	Yes	Yes	Carnivores, rodents	Woolsey and Van der Loos, 1970
Orientation columns	V1	Yes	Yes	Carnivores, rodents, primates	Hubel *et al.*, 1977
Ocular dominance columns	V1	Yes	Yes	Carnivores, primates	Hubel *et al.*, 1977
Blobs	V1	Yes	Yes	Primates (and perhaps some carnivores)	Horton, 1984; Hendrickson, 1985; Murphy *et al.*, 1990
Stripes	V2	Yes	Yes	Primates	Horton, 1984; Hendrickson, 1985
Monaural and binaural columns	A1	Yes	Yes	Carnivores, rodents	Abeles and Goldstein, 1970; Imig and Adrián, 1977; Imig and Brugge, 1978

Callosal and ipsilateral cortico-cortical columns/patches	Frontal and parietal cortex	Yes	Yes	Primates	Jones *et al.*, 1975; Goldman and Nauta, 1977; Goldman-Rakic and Schwartz, 1982
Patches	Entorhinal cortex	No	Yes	Primates	Hevner and Wong-Riley, 1992
Extracortical					
Striasomes	Caudate/putamen	Yes	Yes	All mammals	Graybiel and Ragsdale, 1978
Glomeruli	Olfactory bulb	Yes	Yes	All vertebrates	Golgi, 1874; Allison, 1953
Barreloids	Thalamus	Yes	Yes	Rodents (and probably carnivores)	Belford and Killackey, 1979
Barrelettes	Brainstem	Yes	Yes	Rodents (and probably carnivores)	Belford and Killackey, 1979
Unnamed units	Superior colliculus	No	Yes	Primates	Ramon-Moliner, 1972

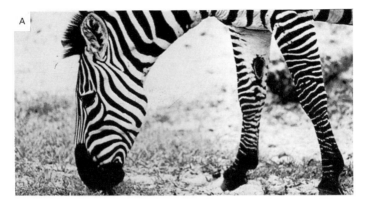

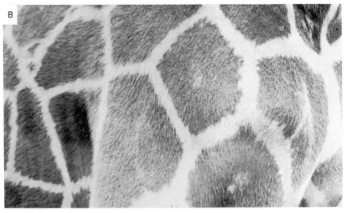

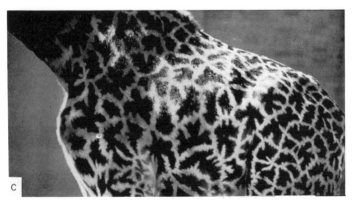

role for modules has been proposed in everything from evolution to neural computation), modular arrangements are actually quite variable among mammalian species. Just to give a couple of examples, ocular dominance columns are present in the visual cortex of Old World monkeys, but are absent in several New World monkeys that have been examined, even though these different primates have otherwise similar visual systems and binocular capabilities (Hendrickson, 1985). Likewise, barrels are found in the somatic sensory cortex of many mammals, but are not present in other, sometimes closely related species (Woolsey *et al.*, 1975). The reasons for these differences among animals are obscure. Suffice it to say that such variation among species tends to confound the idea that a modular organization reflects some functional imperative of cortical operation. By the same token, the proposed rationales for modular patterns – evolutionary, computational or otherwise – remain weak. Lots of animals (and lots of brain regions) just do not have this sort of organization, and yet their brains work just as well and achieve the same behavioral purposes as those in species that do have modules of a particular class.

Figure 2.2 shows similar modular patterns in another mammalian epithelial derivative, the fur (remember that the brain develops from an epithelial sheet, making this comparison less far-fetched than it might seem). The markings on the fur and skin of animals force one to think, by analogy, about the possible purposes of modularity in the brain. Skin and fur markings are so striking that it is natural to assume that they

Figure 2.2. Markings on the skin and fur of mammals have many of the same formal characteristics as the spots, swirls and stripes found in the mammalian brain. It is instructive to think of the origins of these different arrangements when considering the significance of the striking patterns in these two different derivatives of the embryonic epithelium. (From Stevens, 1974.)

must reflect some fundamental function of the integument. The major purposes of the skin, however, are temperature control, water regulation, and protection from infection. In fact, zoologists have often found it rather hard to decipher the role of particular animal markings. Such patterns are sometimes used for camouflage or sexual attraction, but more often than not it is difficult to say just why they are there (see, for example, Cott and Huxley, 1940). Much the same can be said of the modular organization of the brain.

Nevertheless, from the point of view of developmental neurobiology, the modular organization of some brain regions in some species has been, and will continue to be, of tremendous value. Because modules are *visible*, they show at a glance how some aspects of brain circuitry are arranged; they can also indicate which circuits are particularly active (see Lecture IV and Riddle *et al.*, 1993). And since many classes of modules can be counted, they provide a means of assessing the strategy of cortical development with respect to complex circuitry. For instance, monitoring the development of such circuits should indicate whether they are added progressively to the brain, whether they are selected from an initial excess, or whether there is some other way the brain establishes an appropriate number of iterated processing units.

The development of modular circuitry

Figure 2.3 illustrates the several possibilities that come to mind in thinking about such questions. Each circle represents a region of the brain – the cortex, for example – at birth (left) and in maturity (right). The first possibility is that the developing brain uses an essentially static strategy for the generation of modular patterns, in which the full complement of circuitry is elaborated at the outset. In this scenario, further development involves only a proportionate growth of modular elements, like the inflation of a balloon with spots on it: the

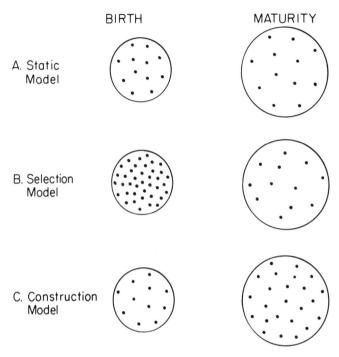

Figure 2.3. Three models of how complex iterated circuits might develop in the mammalian brain (see text for explanation).

number of modules would not change in any interesting or substantial way. A second possibility is what might be called the selectionist model. In this case, there is an excess of complex circuits early on; then, through a process of selection, some of these circuits are eliminated so that the animal ends up with a mature set of modular circuits smaller than the set it began with (see Lecture I). A third possibility is that the brain begins with fewer circuits and adds them progressively as it matures to suit the changing needs of the animal.

We have attempted to distinguish among these alternatives in two regions of the brain. Of course, not all columnar circuitry is appropriate for this kind of analysis. Take, for example, the barrels in the somatic sensory cortex of rodents (and a number of other mammals) that I discussed in Lecture I. Barrels cannot change in number during the course of development because they are isomorphically related to particular sensory specializations in the periphery. Each of the barrels of posterior–medial barrel subfield (the representation of the whiskerpad), for instance, corresponds to one of the large whiskers on the face called the mystacial vibrissae (Woolsey and Van der Loos, 1970). Similarly, the barrel-like structures in the paw representations correspond to the digital and palmar pads on the forepaw and the hindpaw (Dawson and Killackey, 1987). Because the animal has the same number of whiskers and digits when it is born and when it dies, there is no reason to expect any change in the number of these entities – and none is seen (e.g., Riddle *et al.*, 1992). Perhaps one should consider modular arrangements of this kind a special category (see Purves *et al.*, 1994).

Most modular circuits in the brains of mammals, however, are *not* tied isomorphically to a peripheral structure, e.g. the blobs in the monkey visual cortex. Blobs are repeating elements a couple of hundred μm in diameter that can be seen quite easily by means of cytochrome oxidase histochemistry (see Figure 2.1B) (Horton, 1984; Hendrickson, 1985). The function of blobs, as that of other modules, is not really clear. Microelectrode recordings, however, show that blobs are enriched in cells that respond selectively to wavelength (Livingstone and Hubel, 1984); and blobs interconnect specifically to the thick and thin stripes in area 17 (see Figure 2.1B) (Livingstone and Hubel, 1987). There is no doubt, then, that blobs are functionally important circuits, although exactly what they do remains a mystery. But there are no specializations within the retina that correspond to blobs in the way that specific whiskers correspond to cortical barrels.

When A-S. LaMantia and I counted the number of blobs in the visual cortex of newborn and adult monkeys, we found no significant difference between the number determined at birth and the number in maturity: although the blobs grew substantially (more, apparently, than the surrounding cortex), the generation of these entities was largely complete by birth (Purves and LaMantia, 1993). I should perhaps point out that the rhesus monkey is born in a remarkably mature state, as those of you who have dealt with these animals will know. Nonetheless, some brain development in this species certainly occurs postnatally; for instance, the rhesus brain nearly doubles in weight between birth and maturity, and the visual cortex increases in area by about 16% (op. cit.). Even though blobs are not isomorphically tied to any peripheral structure (and so, in principle, could change in number during maturation), the model that seems to fit this case best is the static one (see Figure 2.3).

The mouse pup, unlike the newborn rhesus monkey, is quite immature; mice, then, provide a longer span of postnatal time in which to study brain growth. The options in rodents are limited, however; the only class of telencephalic modules that mice are known to possess (other than barrels) is olfactory glomeruli (see Figure 2.1E). If one takes coronal sections through the olfactory bulb – as Camillo Golgi did in 1874, not far from here in Pavia – it is apparent that the bulb is characterized by small spheres of elaborately developed neuropil that cover its entire surface (Figure 2.4). Golgi named these structures glomeruli. In some respects, glomeruli are structurally similar to the barrels that I discussed in Lecture I; like many barrels, they consist of a rind of cells in Nissl-stained sections that surround a central core of specialized neuropil (cf. Figure 1.8). But unlike barrels, glomeruli (as blobs) are

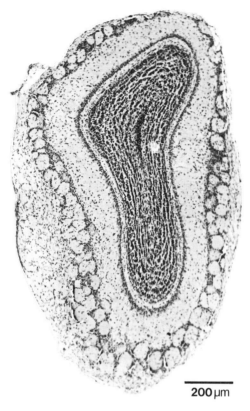

200 μm

Figure 2.4. Coronal section through an adult mouse olfactory bulb showing the pattern of glomeruli (cresyl violet stain). Small spheres of neuropil outlined by a more densely staining rind of neurons that has evidently been excluded from the glomerular center are characteristic of all mammalian (and many other) olfactory bulbs. Such units apparently represent regions of neuropil in which special classes of axonal and dendritic branches have grown to a much greater degree than in the surrounding brain. (From Pomeroy *et al.*, 1990.)

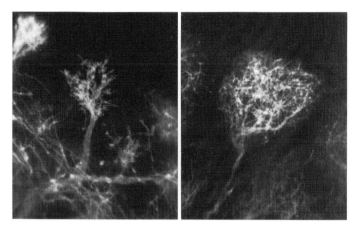

Figure 2.5. Photomicrograph of mitral cells visualized by retrograde fluorescence (Di-I) labeling from the lateral olfactory tract. Each glomerulus represents the efflorescence of the apical dendrite of several mitral cells, which are in turn innervated by afferent sensory axons and numerous interneurons. Each glomerulus, then, is a center of intense neuropil growth. (Pomeroy *et al.*, 1990.)

not tied isomorphically to a particular sensory structure. They are, therefore, free to change, and thus to reveal the developmental strategy that applies to such telencephalic circuitry.

Figure 2.5 shows glomeruli in the same orientation as Figure 2.4, but at higher magnification and stained with a different technique. In this case, the glomeruli have been made visible by applying the lipophilic reagent Di-I to the axons that leave the bulb, thus retrogradely labeling the major efferent neurons (called mitral cells) (Pomeroy *et al.*, 1990). Mitral cells are similar to the Purkinje cells in the cerebellum, or to the layer V pyramids in the cerebral cortex in that they provide the major output of the system. Their apical dendrites run to the surface where, as shown in Figure 2.5, there is a tremendous efflorescence of the secondary and higher order branches. Each glomerulus in the mouse receives at least several apical dendrites from different mitral cells. These branches are innervated by afferents arising from the olfactory epithelium, and in about equal measure by numerous interneurons that run in the plane of the bulbar surface. As with all the other modules I have alluded to, the function of glomeruli is not known; clearly, however, they are the major processing circuits in this first station for the analysis of olfactory information. More importantly, they can be readily observed and counted.

In mice we could develop the techniques to undertake a type of experiment that simply was not feasible to develop for primates: observing the number and arrangement of modules at different times in the *same* animal as it grew to maturity (LaMantia and Purves, 1989; LaMantia *et al.*, 1992). The methods that allowed us to watch complex brain circuits develop over time are of interest, since this approach could be used for a variety of other developmental studies. We were prepared to undertake this work as we had recently been observing the stability of innervation over periods of up to several months in the peripheral nervous system (see Purves and Voyvodic, 1987). Much the same approach could be used to monitor the development of identified modules in the olfactory bulb. A mouse was placed on the stage of a modified microscope, the dorsal surface of the bulb exposed, and an image made and stored in a computer disk file (Figure 2.6A). The animal was then allowed to recover, and to grow up over some interval. We later examined the same animal again to see how the number and configuration of glomeruli had changed. The only significant technical difference in the newer work is that we used a confocal microscope instead of a low-light level video camera because of the confocal microscope's greater ability to reveal structures like glomeruli that are embedded in the substance of the brain (LaMantia *et al.*, 1992).

Even with a confocal microscope, however, glomeruli, or other modular circuits must be made visible with a stain or by some other trick. For this purpose, we used a vital fluorescent dye (called RH414). A small hole was drilled in the bone over the olfactory bulb, which was superfused with sterile solution beneath a glass coverslip; the dura was left intact to preserve the underlying brain from subsequent scarring (Figure 2.6B). The glomeruli in the exposed portion of the bulb were stained transiently by the application of a low concentration of the fluorescent dye to the dura for several minutes. The dye was then removed by washing with additional Ringer's fluid, and observations made through the dura with the confocal microscope. In this way, we could image a fairly large patch of the brain surface and record the arrangement of a large number of identified glomeruli. Figure 2.7 shows a video image reconstructed with the confocal microscope; the fluorescent (lighter) objects are the glomeruli.

When we examined the animal again after an interval of further development, we had two choices. We could either repeat the entire *in vivo* process just described, or we could, as we usually chose to do, make a permanent record by sacrificing the animal, removing the dorsal surface of the bulb and staining it with an ordinary histological reagent such as Sudan Black. This latter strategy proved more convenient because then we could examine the bulb at leisure, rather than being limited to a few minutes of observation in the living animal.

The result of a representative experiment is shown in Figure 2.8. Remember that the object of the exercise was to compare the same brain over time with respect to the number and arrangement of developing modules. On the left is an initial observation made *in vivo*; on the right is the same view 2 weeks later. Several things are different. In the first place, the bulb has grown: thus, to image the same set of glomeruli 2 weeks later (which is a substantial period of development for a mouse), we had to include a bigger surface area. Second, all of

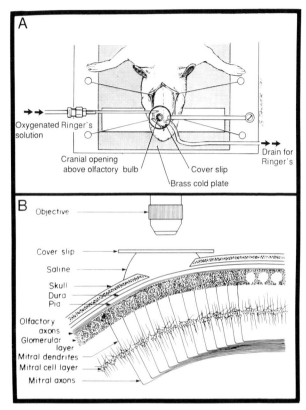

Figure 2.6. *In vivo* imaging of the mouse olfactory bulb. (A) A mouse pup is anesthetized, the head stabilized, and a circle of bone about a millimeter in diameter is then removed to expose the dura overlying the bulb. (B) The relative positions of the dura, arachnoid, pia, nerve fiber layer, and glomerular layer are indicated in a more detailed schematic of the mouse olfactory bulb prepared for vital imaging. To stain glomeruli, the exposed dorsal surface of the bulb, still covered by the dura, is briefly treated with a vital fluorescent dye. *In vivo* images of the glomerular layer are acquired with a laser-scanning confocal microscope. (From LaMantia *et al.*, 1992.)

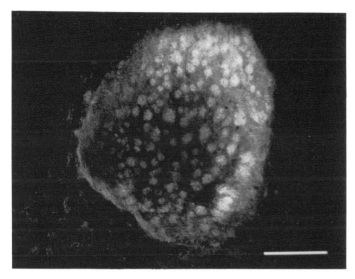

Figure 2.7. Confocal video image of the dorsal surface of a 5-day-old mouse olfactory bulb obtained after fluorescence staining *in situ*; the bright spots are the olfactory glomeruli. In this view, anterior is up and lateral to the left. The fluorescent staining of glomeruli fades within a few hours and disappears within 1–2 days. Scale bar = 250 μm. (From LaMantia *et al.*, 1992.)

the glomeruli present initially are still evident. As in the case of blobs in the visual cortex, there was no evidence for any loss of these complex circuits during maturation. Indeed, there were no exceptions to this rule among the nearly 900 identified glomeruli followed in the animals we monitored. Third, the glomeruli are larger. Like blobs in the monkey visual cortex, the individual circuits grow substantially. But, the point I want to draw your attention to is that new glomeruli (indicated by the plus signs) have been added in the interstices between the existing elements. And, the longer we waited, the greater the

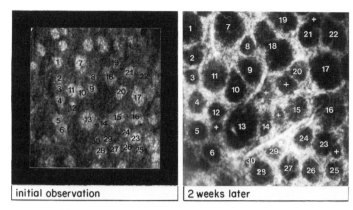

Figure 2.8. Example of the pattern of olfactory glomeruli observed in a mouse a few days after birth (left) and again 2 weeks later (right). The left panel shows the initial image obtained *in vivo*; the right panel shows the final pattern observed after staining the fixed bulb with Sudan Black. Numbers indicate corresponding glomeruli; +s indicate glomeruli added during the interval between observations (see text for further explanation). (From LaMantia *et al.*, 1992.)

number of these newly formed units we saw (LaMantia and Purves, 1989; LaMantia *et al.*, 1992).

Figure 2.9 plots the age of mice against the number of glomeruli in the olfactory bulb to show the full scope and duration of this phenomenon. The absolute number of glomeruli in the mouse bulb is about 400 at birth and about 1700 in maturity, roughly a four-fold increase; the postnatal increment of glomeruli is, therefore, quite large (see, however, Meisami and Sendera, 1993). Moreover, although most of this circuit addition occurs quite early in the mouse's life, it persists in diminishing degree throughout maturation. Mice become sexually mature at roughly 6 weeks; the addition of glomeruli, however, proceeds for about 10–12 postnatal weeks. Thus, circuit addition in this part of the mouse brain

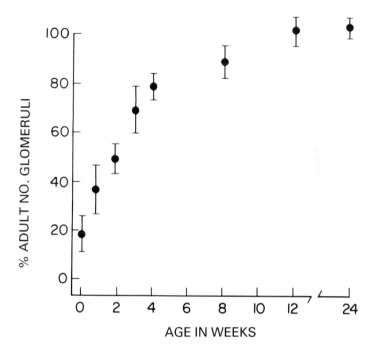

Figure 2.9. Number of glomeruli in the olfactory bulb of developing mice from birth to 24 weeks of age. Each point represents the mean of counts in 10 bulbs from at least 5 different animals; error bars show the standard deviation. Glomeruli are added to the bulb throughout the full period of postnatal maturation. (From Pomeroy *et al.*, 1990.)

goes on over a span that, in a human, would correspond to most of young adult life. These events in the developing bulb are summarized in Figure 2.10, which shows representative computer reconstructions of the olfactory bulb at various ages. In adult mice the arrangement of glomeruli remains stable over time (La Mantia *et al.*, 1992).

Let us return, then, to the possibilities that I outlined on pp. 30–31 (see Figure 2.3). Not surprisingly, the static model

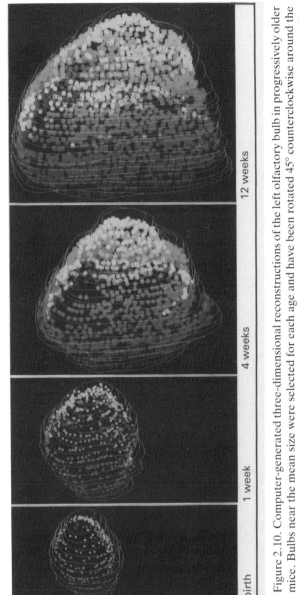

Figure 2.10. Computer-generated three-dimensional reconstructions of the left olfactory bulb in progressively older mice. Bulbs near the mean size were selected for each age and have been rotated 45° counterclockwise around the y-axis; dorsal surface is uppermost, and anterior to right. The glomeruli observed in each section are represented by circles of the same size, scaled to the actual mean diameters at the ages indicated. (From Pomeroy *et al.*, 1990.)

birth 1 week 4 weeks 12 weeks

applies in those instances in which the modular arrangement of cortex is isomorphically related to peripheral sensory structures (e.g., barrels and whiskers in the rat). For blobs in the monkey visual cortex, the static model also appears to describe the way the postnatal brain develops, although here the conclusion is limited by the relative maturity of the rhesus monkey at birth. In neither case is there evidence for an excess of modular circuitry that is subsequently reduced (i.e., the model of Darwinian selection). Finally, in the olfactory bulb, modular circuitry is clearly added for the full period of postnatal maturation. These results in the bulb show that at least some regions of the mammalian brain have the ability to add new units of circuitry for much of early life; and, in all cases, these modular circuits continue to enlarge throughout the period of postnatal maturation.

Conclusion

In Lecture I, I discussed the growth of the brain in relation to the differential growth of maps. In this Lecture I have focused more specifically on the development of the modular elements found within many of these maps. Despite a lot of effort, neurobiologists really do not know why the brain is often organized in a modular fashion. Although the function of modules is an interesting puzzle in its own right, such circuitry provides a fine opportunity for the developmental neurobiologist interested in assessing the strategy of circuit formation, simply because some modular circuits can be seen and counted. The introduction of increasingly sophisticated non-invasive technologies (see, for example, Blasdel and Salama, 1986; Raichle, 1986; Bartfeld and Grinvald, 1992) should make direct evaluation of the development of modular circuitry much more practical in the foreseeable future. The studies done so far indicate that the prolonged growth of the postnatal brain is accompanied by the persistent growth, and, in some cases addition, of complex neural circuitry.

Lecture III

Trophic interactions

In the first two lectures, I discussed brain growth in terms of maps and modules, both macroscopic units of organization measured in hundreds of microns, millimeters, or even centimeters. In this lecture I would like to consider the growth of the brain from the microscopic perspective of the cellular elements that make up these larger entities, and, in particular, the role of trophic interactions in neuronal growth.

Qualitative and quantitative accuracy of neural connections

One major purpose of neuronal interactions during development is to establish *qualitatively* accurate interconnections, i.e., appropriate synapses between the major classes of nerve cells. Since the work of J. Langley in the 1890s, neuroscientists have acknowledged that such qualitative accuracy depends upon 'chemoaffinity' – i.e., the mutual recognition of extracellular and surface markers among pre- and postsynaptic partners (Langley, 1895, 1897). Langley studied this phenomenon in the peripheral autonomic system; chemoaffinity was rediscovered and its understanding greatly advanced, some 50 years later by R. Sperry's work in the retinotectal system (Sperry, 1963). Although neurobiologists have long since agreed that the qualitative accuracy of innervation is based on intercellular recognition, no one yet understands the molecular basis of this process (see, however, Suzue *et al.*, 1990; Donoghue *et al.*, 1992; and Kaprielian and Patterson, 1993, for interesting new approaches).

A second, equally important purpose of neuronal inter-actions vis-à-vis synaptogenesis is to establish *quantitatively* accurate connections. This goal is less frequently mentioned, and relatively few neurobiologists would, in all probability, state this as a fundamental purpose of such interactions. Nonetheless, there is a good deal of evidence that this is the case. Moreover, I want to persuade you that quantitative accuracy of neural connectivity is especially relevant to the issues at hand, namely the mechanisms underlying postnatal brain growth, the role of activity in this process, and the way information is permanently stored in the maturing brain.

Getting the numbers right

Quantitative accuracy of synaptic connections means insuring that the correct number of axons and terminals contact each target cell, and that an appropriate number of target cells is innervated by each axon. Two terms are particularly useful in thinking about these processes, namely divergence and con-vergence (Figure 3.1). Divergence refers to the number of different target cells innervated by each axon; convergence refers to the number of different axons that innervate each target neuron.

Perhaps the reason why people have not paid more atten-tion to convergence and divergence in brain development is simply that the significance of these phenomena is not always obvious. In the case of qualitative accuracy, it is clear that for any part of the nervous system to work properly, neurons of one class have to get to, and innervate, appropriate neurons of another class. The significance of quantitative accuracy can be appreciated in the organization of relatively simple parts of the nervous system, although it is not so apparent in the brain. Consider, for example, the innervation of skeletal muscle. In muscle, the degree of divergence (that is, the number of muscle fibers innervated by each axon, a collection referred to

A   Divergent innervation   **B**   Convergent innervation

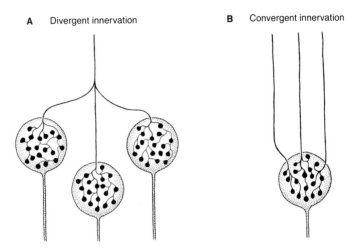

Figure 3.1. Divergent and convergent innervation. (A) Each nerve cell axon usually innervates many target cells (which might be effector cells like muscle fibers and gland cells, or other neurons). This one-to-many relationship is called divergent innervation. (B) From the postsynaptic perspective, each target cell may be innervated by a variable number of different neurons. This relationship is called convergent innervation. Modulation of divergence and convergence by the control of neuronal growth has a major influence on the function of neural pathways. (From Purves, 1988.)

as the 'motor unit') varies from muscle to muscle (Burke, 1983). In small muscles used for delicate movements, such as the lumbrical muscles in the hand, the motor units are small. This arrangement allows the fine, graded responses necessary to pick up a pencil and write, for example. Conversely, in a muscle like the gluteus maximus, the motor units are much larger, consistent with the less delicate function of that muscle. Thus the degree of divergence in the system (reflected in the size of the motor units) has obvious functional consequences. A similar argument can be made for sensory systems, which use more neurons with smaller receptive fields when the perceptual task is a demanding one. There are many more mechanosensory endings in the fingertips, for example, than in the skin of the forearm. And, as in muscle, the endings of each neuron are distributed in a smaller area of the target tissue, in this case providing smaller receptive fields on the fingertips for the finer discrimination that manipulation requires.

The functional significance of convergence can also be appreciated in the peripheral nervous system. Each skeletal muscle fiber is innervated in maturity by a single motor axon. As a consequence, the safety factor of the neuromuscular junction is high: each time the presynaptic axon fires, the postsynaptic muscle cell fires. The situation is quite different for a motor neuron in the spinal cord, where thousands of different inputs converge to innervate each target cell. Accordingly, the synaptic contribution of each presynaptic axon is quite small: instead of being measured in millivolts, the postsynaptic response to each one of these many inputs is measured in microvolts. As a consequence, many axons must be active more or less synchronously to drive the postsynaptic cell to threshold, or to modulate its ongoing activity significantly. In short, different degrees of convergence, just as different degrees of divergence, have profound functional consequences.

The importance of target cell geometry in quantitative accuracy

How then are different values of convergence and divergence set during neural development? Let me explore this question by briefly discussing work we carried out in autonomic ganglia to examine the governance of convergence. This venue, like muscle, has the advantage of organizational simplicity, enabling one to discern the rudiments of an answer that is

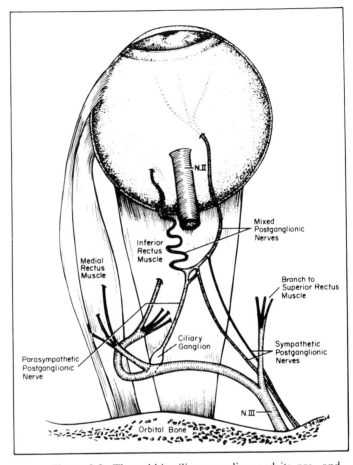

Figure 3.2. The rabbit ciliary ganglion and its pre- and postganglionic nerves. Simple peripheral systems such as this can sometimes reveal principles of organization difficult to discern in the much more complex central nervous system. (From Johnson and Purves, 1981.)

obscured by the sheer complexity of the central nervous system.

The ciliary ganglion in the rabbit is a collection of about 400 parasympathetic nerve cells located in the orbit (Figure 3.2). These neurons have more or less the same function: they are cholinergic cells that run in the postganglionic ciliary nerves to innervate the constrictor muscle of the iris. (It is the constrictor muscle that reacts when a bright light is shone in the eye, causing the pupil to 'narrow'.) These 400 nerve cells are innervated in turn by about 40 preganglionic neurons that reside in the Edinger Westphal nucleus of the brainstem and which reach the ganglion via the third cranial nerve.

Given this arrangement, one can determine precisely, and relatively easily, the degree of preganglionic axonal convergence onto particular ganglion cells. This approach involves impaling the target neurons with a microelectrode and stimulating, in a graded fashion, the axons of the preganglionic nerve (Figure 3.3A; Johnson and Purves, 1981; Purves and Hume, 1981). In the examples shown in Figure 3.3B, the intensity of stimulation to the preganglionic nerve was gradually increased so that more and more preganglionic axons were recruited to fire. In this way, we could measure the postsynaptic response, which occurs (by design) in the refractory period of an antidromic action potential. For the neuron shown in the upper panel, there is a single all-or-nothing response. That is, stimulating the nerve either fails to elicit a response when the stimulus strength is below a certain level, or elicits a full-blown synaptic response when above this level. No matter how many times the trial was repeated (about six are shown), the synaptic response was always unitary, increasing from zero to a maximal value without any intervening steps. This type of response is diagnostic of a target nerve cell that is innervated by a single preganglionic axon.

The lower panel in Figure 3.3B, in contrast, shows a cell with a number of different steps in the postsynaptic response.

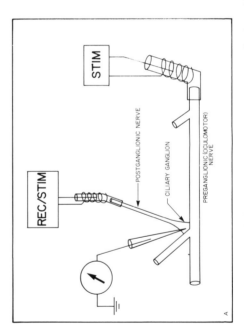

Figure 3.3. Determining convergence among neurons in the rabbit ciliary ganglion. (A) Diagram of the experimental arrangement used to ascertain the number of different axons that innervate each target nerve cell. (B) Incremental responses to preganglionic stimulation. See text for explanation. (From Johnson and Purves, 1981.)

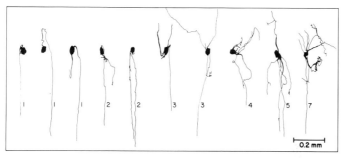

Figure 3.4. The number of axons innervating representative ciliary ganglion cells in adult rabbits. Neurons studied electrophysiologically and then labeled by intracellular injection of horseradish peroxidase have been arranged in order of increasing dendritic complexity. Comparison of the number of innervating axons (indicated by the number to the right of each ganglion cell axon) and neuronal architecture shows a strong correlation between dendritic geometry and input number. (After Purves and Hume, 1981.)

Upon repeated trials, four steps could be counted in the postsynaptic response; this was, therefore, a nerve cell innervated by four different axons. Using this method, we could determine the degree of preganglionic convergence onto a large sample of these relatively simple target neurons. In the central nervous system, the degree of convergence is in most instances vastly greater (up to about 100 000 or more), rendering this approach impractical.

Following such electrophysiological measurements, we injected each nerve cell with a marker to determine its dendritic architecture. There is a range of neuronal geometries in these ganglia, which turns out to be quite important for understanding how convergence is determined. Figure 3.4 shows ten cells from a large sample of neurons that R. Hume and I studied, ordered according to increasing dendritic complexity (Purves and Hume, 1981; Hume and Purves, 1981).

About one-third of the cells in the ganglion lack dendrites altogether, but other neurons have as many as seven or eight primary dendrites. The numbers beside each axon indicate the degree of convergence determined electrophysiologically (as just described). Note that this value increases in parallel with the dendritic complexity: neurons that lack dendrites are innervated by a single preganglionic axon, whereas neurons with many dendrites are innervated by the largest number of axons. Figure 3.5 shows convergence plotted against the number of dendrites for more than 100 ciliary ganglion cells examined in this way.

The robust relationship between target cell geometry and convergence evident in Figure 3.5 is quite general. Hume and I, and later other collaborators in the laboratory, explored this phenomenon in a number of different ganglia in a variety of mammalian species (Purves and Lichtman, 1985b; Purves, Rubin *et al.*, 1986). The link between geometry and convergence is characteristic of sympathetic and parasympathetic ganglia, and occurs across a range of animals in which homologous ganglion cells differ in geometry. The degree of convergence is always well correlated with dendritic complexity among peripheral neurons, at least in those cases where the arrangement of nerve cells and their innervation are simple enough to allow this kind of examination.

How does this linkage of dendritic complexity and convergence arise? The upper panel of Figure 3.6 presents a selection of neurons from the ciliary ganglia of neonatal animals; the lower panel shows the same set of adult neurons that I described previously, ordered again by geometrical complexity. Two differences are apparent. First, the same overall range of geometrical complexity is present in neonates as in adult animals. The cells are smaller, to be sure (dendrites grow substantially during maturation – see Lecture I and Figure 1.1), but at birth there are already neurons that lack dendrites, and neurons that have relatively complex dendritic

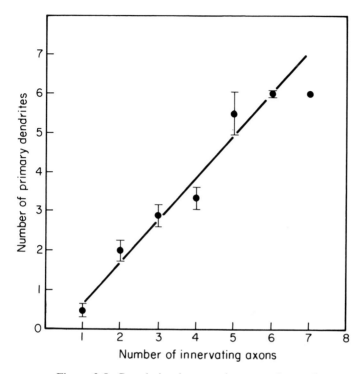

Figure 3.5. Correlation between input number and post-synaptic geometry among rabbit ciliary ganglion cells, using the number of primary dendrites as an index of complexity (see Figure 3.4). Each point represents the mean of measurements on a number of neurons (bars indicate the standard error); the straight line was fitted to the data by a least squares linear regression program and has a slope of about 1. (After Purves and Hume, 1981.)

arborizations. Unlike the situation in adults, however, the degree of convergence is about the same among the ganglion cells in newborn animals. That is, just as many axons, on average, innervate the neurons that lack dendrites as inner-vate the neurons that have complex dendritic trees.

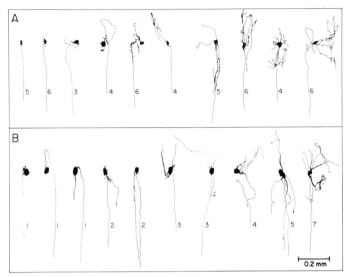

Figure 3.6. Modulation of competition as a result of increasing postsynaptic (dendritic) complexity. (A) At birth, each
neuron in the rabbit ciliary ganglion is innervated by about
the same number of axons (5, on average). (B) By the time
the animal reaches maturity, however, a strong correlation
has been established between geometry and inputs (same
series as Figure 3.4). Comparison of the pattern of innervation at birth and in maturity implies that competitive
interactions between axons innervating the same neuron
are enhanced on neurons that lack dendrites and mitigated
by increasingly complex dendritic arborizations. (After
Hume and Purves, 1981; Purves and Hume, 1981.)

We inferred two points from these observations. First, if a
nerve cell lacks dendrites, then multiple innervation is an
unstable condition. Innervation of the target cell by several
axons is not allowed to persist during the maturation of such
neurons, as if axons limited to the arena of the target cell body
are forced to compete with one another. A second inference is
that when neurons have a significant number of dendrites,

competition between the innervating axons is mitigated. Indeed, to judge from the numbers in Figure 3.6, there is *no net elimination* of inputs during maturation from the surfaces of neurons that have a substantial number of dendrites. The presence of dendritic processes on target neurons apparently forestalls the interaction that forces a reduction of the degree of convergence on neurons that lack dendrites. We have argued, therefore, that one of the major purposes of neuronal dendrites is to modulate competitive interactions between cells in order to set the degree of convergence at an appropriate level (Purves and Hume, 1981; Purves, 1983, 1988). Evidently the mechanism that determines degree of convergence for a particular target nerve cell is the progressive lessening of competition that arises from the presence of increasing numbers of dendrites.

We still do not understand exactly how the presence of dendrites mitigates competition, but the most likely explanation is spatial segregation. When neurons lack dendrites, the competing axons are confined to a relatively small surface area and interact with one another strongly. When the competitors are separated from each other by increasingly complex dendritic branches, the innervating axons interact less strongly and peaceful coexistence becomes permissible. The spatial separation of inputs to the same target cell is, however, a statistical phenomenon, and other explanations remain plausible (see Forehand and Purves, 1984; Forehand, 1985, 1987).

Does setting the value of convergence involve synapse elimination?

Figure 3.7A illustrates the normal evolution of multiple to single innervation during the maturation of cells that lack dendrites. At first glance, this reduction appears to involve the elimination of an initial *excess* of synaptic contacts. In this

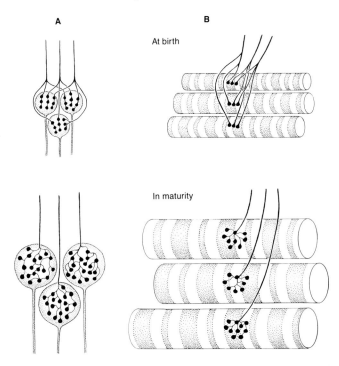

Figure 3.7. Major features of synaptic rearrangement during the first few weeks of postnatal life in the mammalian peripheral nervous system. In ganglia comprising neurons without dendrites (A) and in muscles (B), each axon innervates more target cells at birth than in maturity. In both muscles and ganglia, however, the size and complexity of the terminal arbor on each target cell increase; thus, during early life, each axon elaborates more and more terminal branches and synaptic endings on the target cells it will innervate in maturity. The common denominator of this process is not a net loss of synapses, but the focusing of a progressively increasing amount of synaptic machinery on fewer target cells. (After Purves and Lichtman, 1980.)

particular case, the degree of convergence is certainly reduced and the process clearly entails the removal of some of the synaptic contacts initially made. But note that the outcome does not involve the elimination of an excessive (or 'redundant') number of synapses. The diagram in Figure 3.7A is accurately drawn, being based on electron microscopical evaluation of the numbers of synapses made on ganglion cells that lack dendrites. In fact, the number of synaptic boutons made on target ganglion cells is *smaller* initially than it is in maturity (Lichtman, 1977; Johnson and Purves, 1981). Although the change from multiple to single axon innervation is conventionally called 'synapse elimination', it is a misnomer in the sense that the overall number of synapses is actually increasing during the establishment of an appropriate level of convergence. In reality, each axon gradually makes more and more synapses, albeit on fewer and fewer target cells in this instance.

Muscle fiber end-plates provide another example of a restricted arena within which greater initial convergence will eventually be reduced to one (Figure 3.7B; Redfern, 1970; Brown *et al.*, 1976). And, like the situation in autonomic ganglia, spatial separation of inputs apparently allows the coexistence of multiple innervation (when, for example, there are multiple end-plates on muscle fibers, as in a slow-twitch muscle – Burke, 1983). Moreover, the number and arrangement of synaptic boutons at each end-plate on a muscle fiber are rather similar to ganglion cells (Figures 3.7A and B). Although the transition from polyneuronal to single innervation in muscle appears to involve the elimination of an initial excess, the size and complexity of terminal branches at each end-plate are again increasing (see, for example, Balice-Gordon and Lichtman, 1990, 1993).

Of course, very few cells in the nervous system are like muscle fibers and adendritic ganglion cells, i.e., target cells upon which the degree of convergence is ultimately one. The vast majority of neurons in the central nervous system, as you know, are innervated by hundreds or thousands of inputs and are wonderfully endowed with complex dendrites that identify the major neuronal classes in the brain (stellate cells, pyramidal cells and so on). One of the major reasons for this baroque complexity of central neurons is presumably to set the degree of convergence to a level appropriate for the function of each class of target nerve cell by modulating interactions among the axons innervating the same target cell.

Thus the elimination of synapses, much less the elimination of redundant synapses, is not the cardinal feature of the quantitative accuracy demanded by the developing nervous system. The elimination of some inputs to target cells proceeds on a background of net synaptic gain; moreover, the neuronal interactions leading to elimination are sufficiently forestalled by even a small number of dendrites to insure that there is no net loss of inputs from geometrically complex neurons (see Figure 3.6).

A basis for the interactions that determine convergence

What mechanisms, then, give rise to an apparent competition between innervating axons, such that when they are restricted to the arena of a cell body (or to an end-plate) they interact vigorously with one another? Broadly speaking, the answer lies in a class of interactions between nerve cells referred to as 'trophic'.

By definition, trophic interactions are long-term dependencies of neurons and their synaptic partners manifested in cell survival and neuritic growth; both the phenomena evidently depend on signals provided by target cells to the neurons that innervate them (reviewed in Purves 1977, 1988; Purves *et al.*, 1988). The most compelling evidence for such signaling *vis-à-vis* growth – the more important context for present purposes

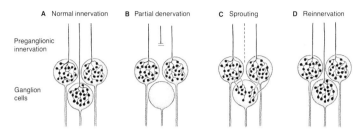

Figure 3.8. Renewed terminal growth and synaptogenesis following partial denervation of target cells. (A) The normal arrangement of innervation among adendritic ganglion cells. (B) When a fraction of the preganglionic axons is cut, some neurons are denervated. (C) Within a few days, the residual (intact) axons send out new terminal branches which innervate the denervated neurons. The fact that the residual terminals are stimulated to grow anew suggests a signal emanating from the denervated cells. (D) When the interrupted axons regenerate, the sprouts give way in favor of the original axons. This phenomenon presumably represents the correction of a quantitative imbalance that occurs when axons with relatively few terminals compete with axons making a surfeit of connections. The entire process is similar to the initial innervation and rearrangement of connections that occurs in normal development. (From Purves, 1988.)

– comes from observations of nerve terminal sprouting and retraction induced by altering the availability of trophic signals. When, in maturity, intact axons are presented with denervated target cells, they respond by sending out additional branches (Figure 3.8). These exploratory sprouts contact the denervated target cells and make functional synapses with them (see, for example, Courtney and Roper, 1976; Roper and Ko, 1978; Brown, 1984). When the cut axons are allowed to regenerate, then the initial arrangement of innervation is largely restored. That is, the newly made sprouts are removed as the original axons re-establish the normal balance

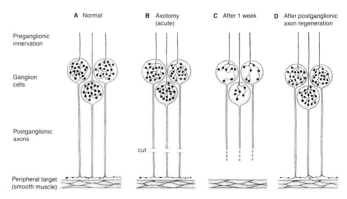

Figure 3.9. Loss of synaptic connections from ganglion cells following interruption of the link between the neurons and their peripheral targets. (A) The postganglionic axons of ganglion cells extend peripherally to innervate smooth muscle or other visceral targets. (B) When the normal connection between ganglion cells and targets is interrupted, the axons distal to the lesion degenerate. (C) Most (but not all) of the synapses on ganglion cells are lost within a week of postganglionic axotomy. (D) The synaptic loss is reversible; full recovery of synaptic function occurs over several weeks, roughly coincident with the regeneration of postganglionic axons to the periphery. This sequence of events indicates an ongoing dependence of ganglionic synapses on a message from the postsynaptic neuron, which depends in turn on the integrity of postganglionic innervation. (From Purves, 1988.)

of connectivity. This sequence of events implies that a signal is provided by the target cells to nearby axons, and that the signal affects growth and the formation of new connections.

A second phenomenon, which is apparently the converse of sprouting, shows further that synapses are *maintained* on target cells by a similar signal or set of signals (Purves, 1975, 1977, 1988). The experimental maneuver in this case is to interrupt the connection between ganglion cells and their peripheral targets (Figure 3.9). Under these conditions, synapses are rapidly lost from the surface of the target ganglion cells: within a few days about two-thirds of the synapses are removed, as can be shown by either electrophysiological or electron microscopical assessment. When postganglionic connectivity is restored by regeneration of the ganglion cell axons to their peripheral targets, then the synapses made on the surfaces of the ganglion cells are regained. As in the case of sprouting, this return to normalcy implies that each ganglion cell broadcasts a message which informs the relevant preganglionic axons that conditions are suitable for innervation. The absence of this signal(s) evidently conveys an opposite message, namely that the ganglion cell is no longer a suitable site for synapse formation and maintenance. As a consequence, synapses are lost.

If this 'axotomy' experiment is carried out on a ganglion in which the nerve cells possess substantial numbers of dendrites, then axon interruption causes dendritic involution, as well as a loss of synapses (Figure 3.10). As with the recovery of ganglion cell synapses, the dendrites of the target cells re-extend to approximately their original length when the preganglionic axon regenerates (Yawo, 1987). Therefore, the mechanism that conveys information about the suitability of the postsynaptic surface for synapse formation also modulates that neuron's dendritic arborization. This dependence of dendritic number and extent on neuronal targets has been nicely confirmed by experiments in which the size of the peripheral target was altered in relation to the number of innervating neurons (Voyvodic, 1989). In these experiments dendritic arborizations were permanently changed by altering the target size.

In short, there is normally a well-controlled *balance* of innervation amongst any given population of axons and their target cells. If a signal (or signals) emanating from the target cell in question is reduced, then there is retraction of the synapses from the surface of the neuron and dendritic shrink-

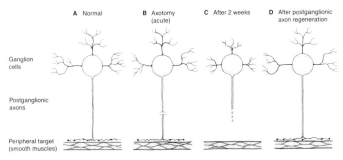

Figure 3.10. Effects of postganglionic axotomy on the dendritic morphology of sympathetic ganglion cells. (A) Normally, neurons in the superior cervical ganglion of mammals have substantial dendritic arborizations. (B) and (C) Within 2 weeks of the cutting of axons that link the ganglion cells to their peripheral targets, the dendritic trees of the neurons shrink by 60%, on average. (D) This effect is reversible. The length and complexity of ganglion cell dendrites are gradually re-established over a period that coincides with the regeneration of postganglionic axons to the periphery. (From Purves, 1988; based on Yawo, 1987.)

age. Conversely, an excess of this signal(s) causes additional synapses to be made, and dendrites to grow. At a macroscopic level, the attainment of this equilibrium sustained by trophic signals must be reflected in the growth and ultimate size of maps, modules, and the brain itself.

The nature of trophic signals

I would like now to discuss briefly the *nature* of such signals. It will come as no surprise to most of you that the best example of a specific trophic signal – the paradigm, if you like – is the molecule of nerve growth factor (NGF) discovered by R. Levi-Montalcini, S. Cohen and V. Hamburger in the late 1940s and early 1950s (Levi-Montalcini, 1987; see also Purves and Sanes, 1987). In the last 40 years, NGF has become one of the best studied molecules in neurobiology, and it is now clear that this agent is a member of a growing family of such molecules, now called the neurotrophins (Barde, 1989; Thoenen, 1991; Loughlin and Fallon, 1993). Nerve growth factor and the several other neurotrophins that have now been well described certainly do not provide all the answers to the phenomenology I have just outlined. A variety of other molecules, from arachidonic acid to nitric oxide, are now being investigated as potential trophic signals; moreover, surface molecules such as receptors and other synapse-specific agents such as neurotransmitters may also be important players in this phenomenology. Nonetheless, NGF and other trophic factors supply some powerful clues about the nature of the signals that modulate the quantitative aspects of neural connectivity, most especially neural growth.

As noted, nerve growth factor has two major effects on neurons that are responsive to it. The first effect is on cell survival. Following uptake at targets and retrograde transport, NGF (or a second messenger activated by it) apparently suppresses the expression of genes that would otherwise lead to cell death (Levi-Montalcini, 1987; Johnson *et al.*, 1989). Although this effect on cell survival is tangential to the present case, it is important to recognize that a major role of NGF and other neurotrophins is to modulate the number of responsive neurons in early embryonic life, and to a much reduced degree in the mature nervous system (see Loughlin and Fallon, 1993).

In addition to the effects of NGF on cell survival, this molecule provides a powerful stimulus to neuritic growth (indeed, the name 'nerve growth factor' is based on this property). It is this effect of the neurotrophins that has been of particular significance for the argument here. The influence of NGF on neurites was recognized from the outset of the remarkable body of work on this agent, and the 'halo effect' of NGF-stimulated growth for several decades provided the standard bioassay for NGF activity (Levi-Montalcini, 1987).

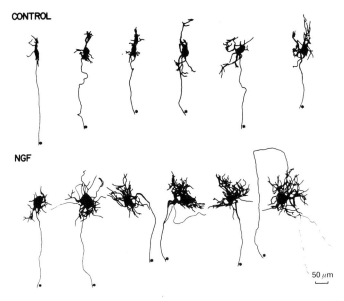

Figure 3.11. Effect of NGF on the dendritic development of superior cervical ganglion cells. Neonatal rats were given a 2-week course of daily subcutaneous injections of NGF; individual neurons from treated and control animals were subsequently filled with the enzyme horseradish peroxidase by intracellular injection to assess their geometry. Neurons from the untreated control animals have shorter and less complex dendrites than ganglion cells from NGF-treated littermates. The number of primary dendritic branches extending from the cell body is also increased. Thus, the size of the dendritic arbors attained by neonatal animals after 2 weeks of NGF treatment is about the same as that attained by untreated animals after 3 months. Asterisks indicate the axon of each cell. (After Snider 1988.)

Further, exogenous NGF administration has long been known to influence the growth of axon terminals (Olson and Malmfors, 1970). More recently, W. Snider (1988) has shown that exogenous NGF also stimulates the dendritic growth of developing neurons in the rat sympathetic system (Figure 3.11).

The diagram in Figure 3.12 outlines the action of NGF on autonomic ganglion cells that are sensitive to it, such as sympathetic neurons. Neurotrophins like NGF are elaborated, at least in a large part, by peripheral target tissues and are taken up by specific receptors on the innervating axons, in this case the axon of a sympathetic ganglion cell. This interaction has a *local* effect on the growth and the extension of the sensitive neurites, providing a plausible basis for the peripheral modulation of connectivity (i.e., the sprouting or terminal retraction at the level of the postganglionic target I described earlier). NGF is retrogradely transported to the parent cell body, where it (or an NGF-dependent second message) modulates the growth of neuronal dendrites (Yawo, 1987; Snider, 1988). At this level, exogenous NGF also has the expected effects on the loss and regeneration of synapses that follow axotomy. If the retrogradely transported NGF that is missing after postganglionic axotomy is artificially supplied by implantation of a pellet that slowly releases the molecule, virtually all of the axotomy effects that I mentioned can be reduced or prevented (Njå and Purves, 1978). Evidently, the ganglion cells themselves supply a further trophic signal that informs more proximal neurons in the pathway about the suitability of the ganglion cell surface for synapse elaboration and maintenance. This additional trophic signal is almost certainly not nerve growth factor, but is apparently under its control; another trophic factor presumably plays the same general role at the level of the ganglion that NGF plays at the peripheral target. In short, at every link in the concatenation of neurons between the central nervous system and the

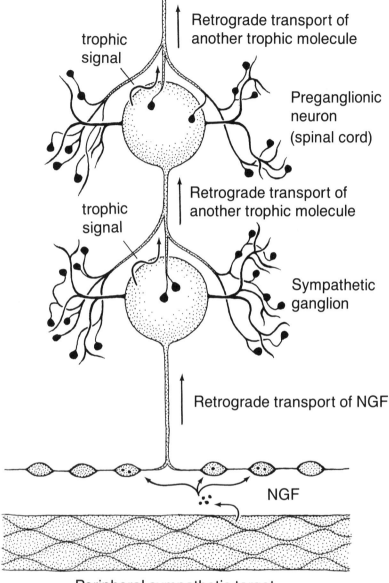

Retrograde transport of
another trophic molecule

trophic
signal

Preganglionic
neuron
(spinal cord)

Retrograde transport of
another trophic molecule

trophic
signal

Sympathetic
ganglion

Retrograde transport of NGF

NGF

Peripheral sympathetic target

periphery, such signals exert the same modulatory control over the growth of nerve cell processes and synapses that NGF demonstrably provides at the most peripheral level.

Conclusion

To summarize the major points that I have made in this lecture, there is a prolonged rearrangement of synaptic connectivity in early life. The primary purpose of this process, I have argued, is not to winnow redundant synapses, but

Figure 3.12. Summary of trophic linkages that coordinate the innervation of targets and central neurons. Neurotrophins such as NGF are elaborated by peripheral targets and interact with specific receptors on the axon terminals of innervating neurons. At this level, trophic molecules modulate the branching of axon terminals by local action; increased availability causes the growth of terminals and decreased availability causes retraction. The trophic signal that reaches the cell body informs each neuron about the degree of its peripheral connectivity, and modulates the dendritic arborization of the parent cell. Because the ganglion cells shown here are in turn the target for preganglionic innervation that arises from neurons in the spinal cord, the elaboration of a second trophic molecule by ganglionic neurons is inferred (ganglion cells do not synthesize or secrete NGF). This second trophic signal evidently controls the neurons that innervate ganglion cells in much the same way that NGF acts on the ganglion cells, namely by local action on the preganglionic terminals that innervate the ganglion cells and by more general retrograde effects on growth after transport to the preganglionic cell bodies in the spinal cord. A further trophic linkage is postulated between the preganglionic neurons and the innervation they receive from higher centers. In this manner, information that initially derives from neural targets can affect the connectivity of an entire pathway. (After Purves, 1986.)

gradually to establish the quantitative accuracy of innervation that is vital to successful neural function (along with the qualitative accuracy achieved by chemoaffinity). Although the developmental loss of some synapses certainly occurs – and despite all the attention focused on 'pruning' and 'selective stabilization' – these regressive processes are hugely overshadowed by the progressive addition of synapses and circuitry. A second point is that competition among axons is strongly modulated by the *arena* in which it transpires. If the site of interaction is limited to a cell body that has no dendrites (or to a muscle fiber end-plate), then the degree of convergence is set at one. If, however, the arena is extended by the elaboration of dendrites, then peaceful coexistence of multiple inputs becomes permissible, presumably by virtue of a spatial segregation of the potentially competing inputs. In simple peripheral systems, however, the addition of dendrites quickly abolishes any *net* elimination of inputs. Finally, the agents of such modulation are signals supplied by neurotrophins and other molecules that play a trophic role. These trophic mechanisms, in the aggregate, regulate the growth of neuropil, which in turn is reflected in the postnatal growth of maps, modules and the brain as a whole.

Lecture IV

Activity

This last talk concerns the most difficult of the issues that I have chosen to discuss, namely the role of electrical activity in the growth of the brain, and in neural development more generally. Perhaps it is obvious that activity *must* play a major role in the development of the nervous system, either directly or indirectly. In its earliest stages, development is largely cell autonomous. Very quickly, however, development comes to depend upon interactions between cells, some of which I reviewed in the last lecture. Once an animal emerges into the world (and indeed well before birth), yet another sort of interaction becomes an essential part of neural development: neural activity – and eventually the postnatal experience that generates much neural activity – modulates the development of the nervous system, and helps to determine the sorts of individuals we become. The importance of experience in neural maturation is self-evident in our own lives. In animals or people who have matured under 'abnormal' circumstances the detrimental influence of altered early experience on adult function and behavior is even more dramatic.

How neural activity *might* lead to information storage

As I remarked in my introduction to these lectures, there are two ways experience could affect our nervous systems – and by experience one really means the electrical activity of nerve cells, since the outside world has no means of influencing the brain other than by generating receptor potentials, action potentials, and synaptic potentials.

The first way that experience could elicit change is by altering the efficacy of circuitry that has already been established. This aspect of experience's influence on the nervous system has received the lion's share of attention over the years, and still does. Most models of learning and memory, for instance, are predicated on the idea that the efficacy of synaptic potentials is changed by the recent history of activity in the nerve cell or circuit at issue. The most recent incarnation of this attractive concept is the intense interest in long-term potentiation (LTP) in the hippocampus as a model for at least some aspects of mammalian memory (Madison *et al.*, 1991; Bliss and Collinridge, 1993). As you know, much current work is focused on understanding LTP in terms of receptors for the neurotransmitter glutamate (op. cit.).

Despite the popularity of the view that memory depends on changing synaptic efficacy, there is another, quite different way that neural activity (read experience) can influence the nervous system, namely by creating new wiring (or by removing existing circuits). That the vertebrate nervous system routinely creates the circuitry to subserve novel behaviors is evident to any student of animal development and behavior. The nervous system of a newborn (or newly hatched) animal produces a repertoire of behavior that has been programmed, in the course of evolution, to deal with conditions and problems the young animal encounters in the world. A striking example is N. Tinbergen's classic study of the fear responses of newly hatched birds (Tinbergen, 1969). This inherent behavioral repertoire clearly depends upon the construction of specific circuitry built up in embryonic life (see, for example, Hamburger, 1977). In short, normal development provides a precedent for constructing circuitry to subserve the behaviors that will, in the normal course of events, be required at various stages of an animal's life.

It is only natural to wonder, then, if the activity generated by different kinds of *individual* (as opposed to species-specific) experience might affect the ongoing elaboration of neural circuitry in postnatal life. Adding further interest to this possibility, as I have emphasized in the preceding lectures, is evidence that modulation of neural growth is a central feature of development. In any event, it is this idea that I want to explore in the final installment of this series. The difficulty arises because there is relatively little experimental work in this domain.

The effects of activity in the developing visual system

The two most important observations on the role of neural activity in development have come from work on the visual system carried out in the 1960s by D. Hubel and T. Wiesel (reviewed in Hubel, 1982, 1988; Wiesel, 1982). Their experiments continue to provide the best indicator of how activity affects neural development, and stand as the Rosetta stone in this domain. Accordingly, the interpretation of this central body of observations should be re-examined frequently.

The visual system, as you know, is organized in a way that is especially advantageous to physiologists: the inputs from the two eyes are kept separate throughout the system until the level of the cortex, where axons related to the right and left eyes come eventually together to innervate target cells in the primary visual cortex. Thus, cortical neurons can be innervated by inputs related to one eye or the other, or to both eyes (Figure 4.1A). The categorization of cortical neurons according to their degree of 'binocularity' provided Hubel and Wiesel with a powerful index of the effect of activity on brain development.

The approach was more or less the same in both their classical experiments: the effects of visual deprivation were assessed by making electrical recordings from single neurons in the cat visual cortex, noting the responses to stimuli presented to one eye or the other. In this way, cortical neurons

(A)

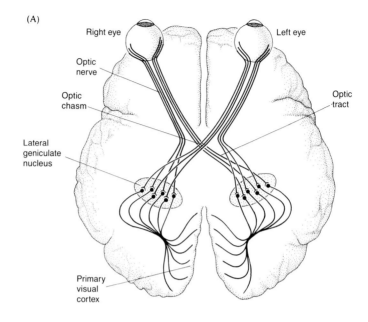

Figure 4.1. Ocular dominance and the effects of monocular deprivation. (A) The visual pathway from the retina to the primary visual cortex. (B) Effect of early monocular closure on the number of cortical neurons driven by each eye. *Upper panel* Normal distribution of binocularity observed in unit recordings from a large sample of neurons in the striate cortex of an adult cat. Cells in group 1 were driven exclusively by the contralateral eye; cells in group 7 by the ipsilateral eye. *Lower panel* Following monocular lid suture (in this case for a period from 1 week after birth until age 2.5 months when the experiment was carried out), no cells could be driven by the deprived (contralateral) eye, although some cells could not be driven by either eye (broken line). (**A** From Purves, 1988; **B** after Hubel and Wiesel, 1962; Wiesel and Hubel, 1963.)

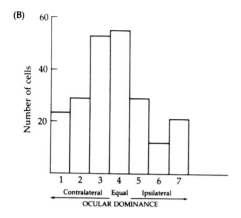

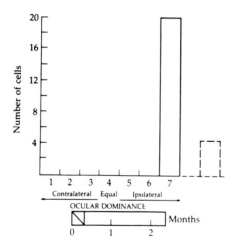

were classified as being dominated by the right eye, the left eye, or both eyes (Figure 4.1B). The resulting 'ocular dominance histogram' differentiates neurons into seven groups, ranging from those responsive only to stimuli presented to the contralateral eye to those responsive only to stimuli presented to the ipsilateral eye; between these extremes are five intermediate groups responsive, in varying degrees, to stimuli presented to both eyes. For a normal cat, the majority of cortical cells fall into categories 2–6; that is, they are responsive to stimuli presented to either eye.

The first experiment involved a reduction of activity in the neurons related to one eye only (Wiesel and Hubel, 1963). Deprivation in early life was achieved by suturing the eyelid shut to reduce retinal activity. The result was a dramatic change in the ocular dominance histogram: neurons that would have been binocularly driven became dominated by the eye that remained open (the contralateral eye in Figure 4.1B). This result showed, quite clearly, that neural activity modulates binocular innervation in the visual cortex.

Most neurobiologists have taken this result to mean that the primary role of activity is to *sustain* (i.e., prevent the loss of) connections already present in the cortex. This idea is often expressed by saying that activity serves to 'validate' or to 'stabilize' appropriate cortical connections, the others being 'pruned' away. A good reason for this consensus is that when visual cortical neurons are tested at the earliest time that responsive neurons in the cortex can be found, the cells already show many of the specific properties that characterize them in adult animals (Hubel and Wiesel, 1963; see also Barlow, 1975). Thus neurons in a newborn cat already have orientation selectivity and other receptive field properties associated with the adult connectivity of the system (although these properties are generally less well defined than in maturity). It seemed reasonable to conclude, therefore, that the intricate cortical connectivity underlying these features is already present at the beginning of visual experience. Accordingly, the primary role of activity was inferred to be a validation and sustenance of the neonatal connections, thus preventing a loss that presumably occurs after monocular deprivation.

The second experiment carried out by Hubel and Wiesel also used the ocular dominance histogram to examine the binocularity of cortical neurons. In this work, however, the amount of visual cortical activity was kept constant; only the synchrony of activity from the two eyes was varied (Figure 4.2; Hubel and Wiesel, 1965). They did this by making newborn animals strabismic, or by alternately occluding one eye and then the other. Animals such as the cat or monkey have frontal eyes and good binocular vision; thus they see largely the same scene with the two retinas (just as we do). Because of the precise somatotopic mapping of the retina (via the geniculate) onto the cortex (see Lecture I), the axons that innervate a binocularly driven cortical cell will normally be active more or less simultaneously, regardless of which eye they are related to. As a result of strabismus or alternating occlusion, however, such cells in the visual cortex come to be driven by one eye or the other, but not by both (Figure 4.2). Thus 'desynchronizing' the activity of the inputs to a target neuron forces one set of axons to lose in a competition with the other set. This outcome implies that the amount of cortical activity *per se* is not terribly important in the development of the visual system. Although the effects of monocular deprivation experiments (see Figure 4.1) *might* be regarded as arising from a reduction of overall activity, simply desynchronizing binocular activity – thus keeping the overall activity of the competitors about the same – yields the same result. This outcome appears to rule out a simple use-dependent explanation. Other experiments have supported this view (e.g., Guillery, 1973; Hubel *et al.*, 1977).

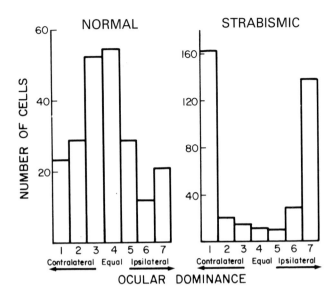

Figure 4.2. Effects of the temporal ordering of input activity on the innervation of neurons in the mammalian visual cortex. Animals with eyes placed towards the front of the head have varying degrees of binocular vision since both eyes see substantially the same scene. Accordingly, corresponding points on the two retinas are subjected to roughly the same spatiotemporal pattern of visual stimuli. This situation can be changed by cutting some of the extraocular muscles, so that the two eyes – now with different directions of gaze – see different scenes. The effects of this procedure were assessed in the cat by recording the responses of individual neurons in the visual cortex to stimulation of one eye or the other, as in Figure 4.1B. In adult cats made strabismic at birth, only about 20% of the neurons in the adult cortex are binocularly driven. Disconjugate gaze desynchronizes the activity of the cortical inputs arising from the two eyes, but does not change the overall activity level. The experimental effect, therefore, is assumed to arise from increased competition among inputs to the same cortical neurons. (After Hubel and Wiesel, 1965.)

An alternative interpretation of the effects of visual deprivation

Despite the prevalence of this interpretation, the results of such desynchronization experiments do not necessarily mean that overall levels of activity are not important in development. Not many years after Hubel and Wiesel's pioneering experiments, people recognized that very, very few of the connections found in the mature visual cortex of the cat are present at birth (e.g., Cragg, 1975). The vast majority of synapse formation still lies ahead for the newborn cat, and indeed for newborn mammals generally (perhaps most especially for humans).

Another view of the role of activity in brain development, therefore, is that *it promotes neuropil growth that would otherwise not occur*. In this conception of the developmental role of neural activity, monocular neurons arise after deprivation not primarily because connections are lost (although some certainly are), but *because large numbers of synaptic connections that would normally have been made by the less active axons fail to grow*. In the 1960s, when Hubel and Wiesel's work on this was carried out, relatively little attention was paid to trophic interactions, competition for trophic factors, or to the growth-related phenomena that I have discussed in these lectures. Not surprisingly, then, these experiments were not considered in such a framework; today they would be. Indeed, very nice work recently carried out here in Pisa addresses directly the role of nerve growth factor in monocular deprivation effects (Maffei, *et al.*, 1992).

Some pertinent observations in the peripheral nervous system

Experiments in the peripheral nervous system support the view that neural activity has a marked influence on neuronal

A   Normal

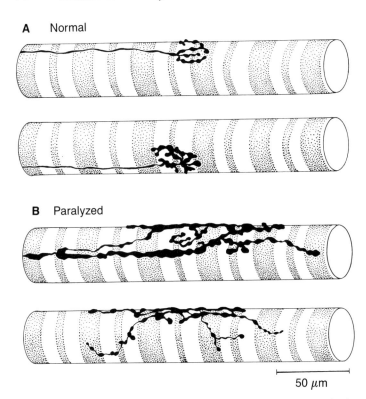

B   Paralyzed

50 μm

Figure 4.3. Renewed growth of motor nerve terminals induced by muscle paralysis in adult mice. (A) Normal terminal arbors at end-plates in a limb muscle, stained by a conventional histological method (zinc iodide-osmium treatment). (B) Terminal arbors on fibers from a muscle treated for 7 days with daily local injections of a neuro-muscular blocking agent. The presynaptic terminals sprout extensively in the absence of postsynaptic activity. See text for interpretation. (After Holland and Brown, 1980.)

growth, and further imply that the agency of this effect is modulation of normal trophic interactions among synaptic partners.

For instance, sprouting of axon terminals occurs in both muscle and adult ganglia when activity is blocked (Brown and Ironton, 1977; Roper and Ko, 1978; Holland and Brown, 1980). This sequence of events was nicely demonstrated for adult muscle fibers by M. Brown and his colleagues some years ago (Brown *et al.*, 1981). If activity is prevented for a few days with a neuromuscular blocking agent, then the motor nerve terminals begin to sprout (Figure 4.3). Furthermore, if activity in developing muscle fibers is prevented by a neuro-muscular blocking agent such as curare or tetrodotoxin, the progression of synaptic rearrangement is stalled (Benoit and Changeux, 1975; Thompson *et al.*, 1979; Brown *et al.*, 1981; Caldwell and Ridge, 1983; see also Jackson 1983). Con-versely, if activity is artificially augmented, the transition from polyneuronal to single innervation is hastened (O'Brien *et al.*, 1978; Thompson, 1983). As I emphasized in the last lecture, neural targets are evidently capable of generating signals that convey the level of their desire to be innervated. The absence of activity appears to augment this signal. Normally, an appropriate level of postsynaptic activity signifies that a suf-ficient level of innervation has been attained; when activity is blocked, target cells are evidently 'fooled' into responding as if they were no longer adequately innervated. At all events, this body of work shows that the activity of synaptic partners in the peripheral nervous system can modulate the growth of the synaptic connections between them.

Another relevant observation in the periphery concerns the arrangement of innervation in autonomic ganglia. When R. Hume and I filled single preganglionic axons with a marker enzyme to examine the distribution of terminals in the rabbit ciliary ganglion, we found that a single axon innervates just a few widely distributed target cells (much like the innervation

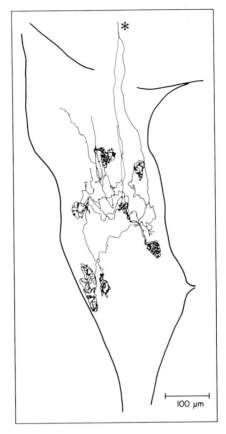

Figure 4.4. Avidity of an innervating axon for a few distributed target neurons within an autonomic ganglion. Tracing shows the arborization of a single labeled axon in a rabbit ciliary ganglion after intra-axonal injection of a marker. The outline shows the size and shape of the ganglion; the asterisk indicates the site at which the axon was injected with horseradish peroxidase. Although the labeled axon ramifies widely, it elaborates many synapses on a few neurons (indicated by clusters of synaptic boutons) scattered among the several hundred potential target cells. The impression that the labeled terminals are sharply confined to a few densely innervated cells has been confirmed by electron microscopy. (From Hume and Purves, 1983.)

of muscle fibers in a motor unit). On each of these target neurons, however, the preganglionic axon made *many* synaptic boutons (Figure 4.4; Hume and Purves, 1983). J. Lichtman (1980) had reached a similar conclusion based on electrophysiological experiments in another ganglion. As I mentioned in Lecture III, the ciliary ganglion is functionally homogeneous: all of the preganglionic axons are cholinergic, and all the ganglion cells have pretty much the same target (the constrictor muscle in the rabbit's eye). In principle, then, *any* preganglionic axon could innervate *any* ganglion cell. Obviously, this is not what happens. Each axon elaborates more and more synapses on only a few target neurons. Why then does this progressive focusing of innervation from an axon onto a few target cells occur?

Lichtman and I suggested a model to account for these observations in the peripheral nervous system (Lichtman and Purves, 1983; Purves and Lichtman, 1985a; see also Purves 1988); the same model could also explain the effects of monocular deprivation on binocularity. The argument supposes that the trophic support provided to innervating axons is dependent upon the simultaneous activity of the pre- and postsynaptic cell (Figure 4.5). This is a Hebbian mechanism, if you like, but applied in a specific context, namely that of trophic interactions. In 1949, the psychologist D. Hebb emphasized the probable importance of conjoint pre- and postsynaptic activity as a mechanism of learning. Since then, many specific mechanisms have been suggested to put flesh on the bones of Hebb's theory. The idea Lichtman and I proposed is that the trophic support from a postsynaptic target neuron to the presynaptic neuron that innervates it will be provided only when both cells are active. In this scheme, less trophic support is provided to a presynaptic cell that is not active in concert with the majority of the synapses on the target neuron, and conversely. The operation of such a rule would cause a transition from a few synapses being made by many axons on a target cell, to many synapses made by a few

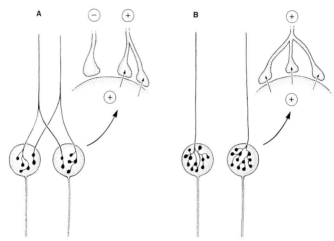

Figure 4.5. Diagram of the linkage envisioned between neural activity and trophic feedback. (A) Initially, ganglion cells that lack dendrites are innervated by several axons (see Lecture III). The assumption of the model depicted here is that acquisition of trophic support depends on simultaneous activity (depolarization) of the pre- and post-synaptic cells (blow-up on right). The number of synaptic boutons initially made by each axon on a given target cell is stochastic. In consequence, whenever an axon with a plurality of terminals on a target cell is active (+), it gains trophic support at the expense of an inactive axon (−) that makes fewer synaptic contacts. Ultimately, the minority terminals are withdrawn from the target cell, and the 'losing' axon elaborates additional terminals on other target cells on which it had the initial advantage. Note that if two axons are consistently active together, they will behave as a single set, just as would multiple endings arising from a single innervating axon. (B) The outcome of such activity-dependent positive feedback among neurons not synchronously active is to concentrate each axon's endings on a smaller number of target cells; those that are active together can, if the activity is synchronized across populations, manifest their common function in macroscopic organization such as the modular cortical patterns described in Lecture II. (From Purves, 1988.)

axons (see Figure 4.5). This rule could also explain why the spatial separation of inputs diminishes their competitive interaction, since depolarization at any given site falls off as a function of the passive electrical properties of the target cell (see Lecture III). Note that the basic mechanism proposed is activity-dependent growth.

Whether this particular mechanism actually operates is, of course, not known. But the operation of *some* mechanism *like* this, i.e., the activity-dependent modulation of trophic interactions, seems essential to explain the phenomenology of synapse formation apparent in muscles, ganglia, and the brain. Hubel and Wiesel's classical observations in the visual system (the effects of monocular deprivation and strabismus), which remain otherwise unexplained at the level of cell biology, can be rationalized in this way. The axons related to the deprived eye fail to grow, whereas axons related to the intact eye grow apace. In the strabismus experiments, activity is normal, as is the growth of the related terminals. The terminals simply prosper on different target cells. The decreased binocularity observed arises from the dependence of trophic support on conjoint pre- and postsynaptic activity (as diagrammed in Figure 4.5). Activity-dependent modulation of neuronal growth thus has the attractive feature of accounting for both the temporal and scalar effects of activity observed in these various experiments in the central and peripheral nervous system. It has the further advantage of explaining all the results so far observed without recourse to any active process of synapse elimination.

There is, of course, another well-known precedent for the hypothesis that the growth of excitable cells is influenced by the amount of their activity. Although neurobiologists do not ordinarily consider the atrophy (and hypertrophy) of muscle cells in relation to the development of the brain, it may be an instructive comparison. Muscle fibers shrink dramatically if they are not innervated. (e.g., Tower, 1939). Moreover, if you have ever had your arm in a cast (or followed the problems of astronauts in a weightless environment), you know that atrophy follows disuse. When a muscle is idle, for whatever reason, its substance tends to diminish; when activity returns, muscle bulk is restored. The effects of activity on cell size are equally apparent in smooth and cardiac muscle, where they have important clinical consequences. Surprisingly, the basis of muscular atrophy and hypertrophy is still not well understood at the cell and molecular level: the link between depolarization, muscle contraction, and growth remains largely obscure (see, for example, Goldberg *et al.*, 1975; Furuno *et al.*, 1990). Nonetheless, these graded activity-dependent changes in muscle show that the amount of ongoing activity modulates the growth of at least some classes of excitable cells.

Neural activity and the growth of the brain

I want now to bring the argument full circle by discussing recent evidence that activity modulates the growth of the brain using as an example the primary somatic sensory cortex that I described in the first of these lectures.

Remember that the somatic sensory map in the rat nearly doubles in area during postnatal development, and that the growth of different regions within S1 is heterogeneous (Riddle *et al.*, 1992). To reiterate, some regions of S1 grow more than others, S1 as a whole grows more than the rest of the neocortex, and the cortical representations of specialized sensors (barrels) grow much more than the intervening (interbarrel) cortex. Could these effects arise from differential neural activity in the various subregions of S1, and might this linkage help to explain our ability to store the effects of experience in a more or less permanent fashion as we grow up?

I mentioned earlier that we had used standard histo-chemical stains to delineate the S1 map and thereby to measure it. I did not discuss, however, what such stains identify, and why they mark most intensely the regions of the somatotopic map that grow the most. These staining methods – succinic dehydrogenase and cytochrome oxidase histochemistry – reveal differences in the distribution of mitochondrial enzymes that are important in metabolism. Succinic dehydrogenase and cytochrome oxidase are located in the cristae of mitochondria, and function in both the citric acid cycle and the electron transport chain to produce the high-energy phosphate bonds on which the life and growth of neurons and other cells depend (e.g., Weibel, 1984; Wong-Riley, 1989). Regions that stain intensely for these enzymes are, therefore, metabolically more active.

Figure 4.6A shows a portion of the rat primary somatic sensory cortex stained for cytochrome oxidase activity, revealing again the obvious difference between the density of the enzymatic reaction product in barrels and in the surrounding interbarrel regions (see Lecture I). Remember that barrels are the regions of S1 that grow the most. In Figure 4.6A you can see that ink has also been injected into the vascular system to visualize the capillary bed. With image processing it is possible to give these ink-filled microvessels sufficient contrast to determine their distribution over large areas automatically (Figure 4.6B). The capillary density is not uniform across S1, but is greater within the regions that stain heavily for mito-chondrial enzymes – the barrels – than in the adjacent, lighter staining regions (interbarrels). Table 4.1 shows a series of measurements in adult rats in which vessel density is ex-pressed as the percentage of the total pixels per unit area occupied by capillaries. There are about 50% more capillaries in the barrels compared to the intervening interbarrel region; and there is about a 20–30% difference between the regions delineated by barrels and the adjacent regions that have no barrels (Riddle *et al.*, 1993). In juvenile animals these differences in microvessel density are even more pronounced, and again accord quite precisely with regional differences in cortical growth. Figure 4.6C indicates that the entire S1 map and its component representations (the 'ratunculus' of Lecture I) stand out because of their greater vascularization compared to the surrounding neocortex.

Such variations in vascular density are not limited to S1 and its barrels, but can be detected for other classes of modules I reviewed in the second lecture. For example, D. Zheng, A-S. LaMantia and I studied this phenomenon in cytochrome oxidase-stained blobs in the monkey cortex (Zheng *et al.*, 1991). We found that blood vessel density in these modules is also about 40% greater than in the surrounding (interblob) cortex. Evidently, the greater metabolic demand of these special regions of the visual cortex – like barrels in the somatic sensory cortex – generates a greater blood supply.

Is there a link between this evidence of regionally different brain metabolism and electrical activity? L. Sokoloff and his colleagues have demonstrated, in a beautiful series of experiments, that most brain metabolism reflects the need to maintain ion gradients across cell membranes (Sokoloff, 1977,

Figure 4.6. Analysis of microvessel distribution in (and around) the primary somatic sensory cortex of the rat. (A) Photomicrograph of ink-filled microvessels and barrels (revealed by cytochrome oxidase staining) in the anterior snout representation. (B) Digitized and processed image of microvessel profiles in (A); lines indicate barrel borders. Such images were used to measure microvessel density in the various regions of S1. (Scale bar = 100 μm.) (C) Overall map of microvessel distribution in cortical layer IV of S1. The average density in each of the major somatic representations within S1 is higher than in the non-barrel S1 regions and the cortex surrounding S1 (Scale bar = 2 mm.) (From Riddle *et al.*, 1993.)

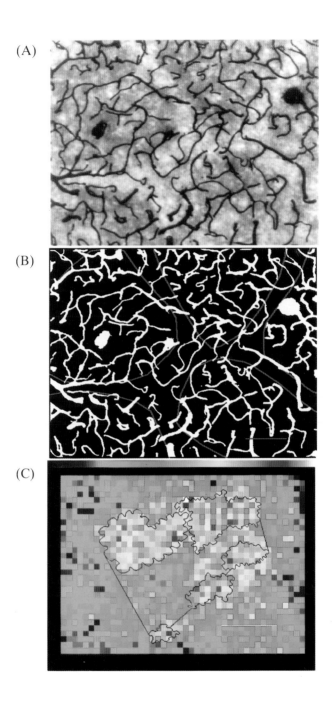

Table 4.1. *Differential distribution of capillaries in the rat primary somatic sensory cortex. (From Riddle et al., 1993.)*

Hemisphere number	Mean blood vessel density (expressed as percent of sampling area)				Percent differences		
	Barrel cortex	Interbarrel cortex	Non-barrel S1 cortex	Peri-S1 cortex	Barrel/ interbarrel cortex	Barrel/ non-barrel S1 cortex	Barrel/ peri-S1 cortex
1	10.2	6.8	8.6	7.4	50	19	38
2	18.2	13.7	15.8	14.1	33	15	29
3	13.0	9.2	11.3	9.4	41	15	38
4	13.5	9.4	11.9	10.3	44	13	31
5	15.9	11.3	14.3	13.4	41	11	19
6	18.2	11.8	15.6	14.8	54	17	23
7	16.6	9.7	13.3	13.7	71	25	21
8	16.1	10.9	12.3	11.1	48	31	45
9	16.9	11.3	13.6	13.7	50	24	23
10	14.6	9.6	11.8	11.0	52	24	33
Mean ± SEM	15.3 ± 0.8	10.4 ± 0.6	12.9 ± 0.7	11.9 ± 0.8	48 ± 3	19 ± 2	30 ± 3

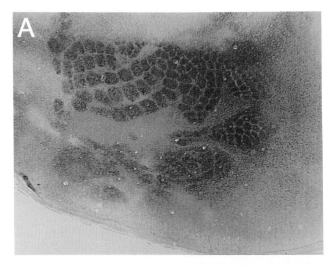

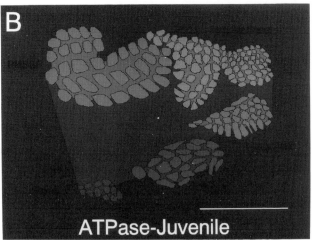

Figure 4.7. Evidence for increased electrical activity of the metabolically more active regions of the rat primary somatic sensory cortex. *Left* (A) Differential distribution of sodium/potassium ATPase in the rodent barrel cortex; barrels in this case are revealed by their greater activity of sodium/potassium ATPase. (B) Grey scale map of ATPase activity across S1 determined by regional densitometry.

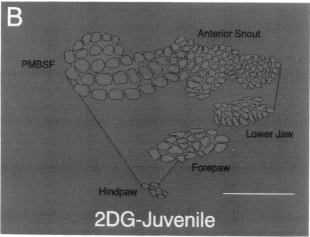

Figure 4.7 (*cont.*). *Right* (A) Differential distribution of 2-deoxyglucose accumulation in the primary somatic sensory cortex of the rat under conditions of normal behavioral activity. (B) Grey scale map of 2-DG accumulation determined by regional densitometry. See text for further explanation. (From Riddle *et al.*, 1993.)

1978, 1979, 1981; Mata *et al.*, 1980). Evidently, about 80% of energy consumption in the adult brain supports the sodium/ potassium exchange on which neural signaling ultimately depends. These facts about energy consumption in the central nervous system suggest that the differential metabolic activity of the cortex is associated with differential electrical activity. We evaluated this implication by looking at the cortical distribution of sodium–potassium ATPase, a membrane-bound enzyme that exchanges Na^+ for K^+. This exchange pump is distributed in the same pattern as succinic dehydro-genase, cytochrome oxidase and blood vessels (Figure 4.7A). The same pattern is observed for radiolabeled deoxyglucose accumulation (Figure 4.7B). Finally, electrophysiological measurements in rat cortex support the idea that the average electrical activity of metabolically active regions like barrels is greater than the activity in regions that are less active meta-bolically. These several lines of evidence all point to the same conclusion: the differential energy consumption of cortical regions reflects systematic differences in their average electri-cal activity. Specialized cortical areas of high metabolic and electrical activity such as barrels are – as I emphasized earlier – the regions that grow most during development (see Lecture I, and Riddle *et al.*, 1992; 1993).

Some caveats

Taken together, these findings support the hypothesis that brain growth is modulated by the differential metabolic and electrical activity of its component parts, an idea we have come to refer to as the 'glow and grow' theory. It must nonetheless be demonstrated by altering activity that this link is indeed a causal one. The task is complicated by the fact that removing peripheral input does not abolish cortical activity, probably because of compensatory changes at several levels of the somatic sensory system (Gutierrez *et al.*, 1993). More-over, it is important to remember that activity can only *modulate* growth, and cannot strictly determine it. At most, neurons completely silenced by removing their normal inputs will continue to grow, but at a reduced level. Perhaps the clearest demonstration of this assertion is the continued growth of autonomic ganglion cells entirely deprived of activity during development by surgical interruption of the nerve that innervates them (the cervical sympathetic trunk; Voyvodic, 1987). Although the absence of activity over the full course of development inhibits the growth of the neurons and their processes by about 35%, in the rat neuronal growth certainly continues in the absence of activity. This outcome is explained, at least in part, by the ongoing support that ganglion cells derive from the targets that they innervate (see Lecture III). In any event, this experiment demonstrates that the effect of activity on neuronal growth, in the periphery at least, is a modulatory one, rather than being an absolute determinant. A number of factors orchestrate the growth of nerve cells, including the trophic support derived from neur-onal targets and a variety of intrinsic neuronal mechanisms that generate growth.

Let me re-emphasize what I take to be the importance of the view that activity modulates neuropil growth, rather than functioning to stabilize synaptic connections, or to help select useful connections from an initial excess. Consider a region of the human brain such as the cortical area that stores infor-mation about the meanings of words (Wernicke's area; Figure 4.8). In the course of growing up – a period of many years in humans – this area, like the rest of the brain, grows. People who are linguistically inclined practice language to a greater degree and accumulate a larger vocabulary than their less verbal peers. On the basis of the evidence outlined here, it seems reasonable to suggest that such prolonged practice stimulates the relatively greater growth of the cells and circuits

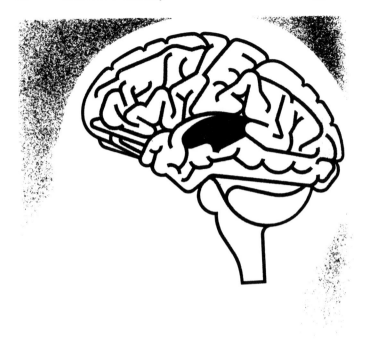

Figure 4.8. Diagram showing Wernicke's area in the human brain. The storage of information about the meaning of words in this region can be explained in terms of circuit construction promoted by neural activity. (After Corsi, 1991.)

of this region. The linguistic (or other) information that the practiced individual retains throughout life is, in this view, a consequence of the further construction of the stimulated neural circuitry. A progressive weakening of the linkage between activity and growth in maturing mammals could explain our diminished ability to learn as we grow older (a fact of psychology referred to as the 'critical period' phenomenon; see Johnson and Newport, 1989, for evidence in respect to learning language). The progressive diminution of brain growth as we mature (see Lecture I) eventually leaves only a low level remodeling as an agent of further structural change in the adult nervous system (e.g., Purves, Hadley and Voyvodic, 1986; Purves *et al.*, 1987). The ability to modify the *efficacy of existing connections* to achieve less permanent changes clearly remains in adult animals, presumably dominating our ability to store new information in maturity.

Conclusion

I have tried to make several general points in these lectures. First, the brain is apparently constructed by the gradual accretion of circuitry, and not by the selection of circuitry from initial excess. This assertion should not be taken to mean that there is no early rearrangement of synapses, or that many synapses are not lost during development. Both phenomena certainly occur. But to focus on synaptic loss is to raise a subsidiary theme of the development of neural circuitry to the status of its driving force. The major theme, in my view, is the growth of the brain, and the vast amount of novel circuitry that this process reflects.

The gradual construction of circuitry, over a period of many years in humans, allows this process to be modulated by neural activity (experience). An increasing body of evidence indicates that electrical activity of the nervous system promotes the growth of brain neuropil, perhaps in much the same way that activity promotes the growth of excitable cells in other systems. Whatever its cellular and molecular basis turns out to be, activity-dependent growth provides a richer and more consistent framework for thinking about neural development than the now popular idea that we start life with an initial excess of connections and then select from this surfeit by competitive mechanisms akin to natural selection. Rather, the brain builds the circuitry it needs during its progress to maturity. Although the vast majority of this construction must arise from developmental programs laid down during the evolution of each species, neural activity can modulate and instruct this process, thus storing the wealth of idiosyncratic information that each of us acquires through individual experience and practice.

Bibliography

Abeles, M. and Goldstein, M.H. (1970) Functional architecture in cat primary auditory cortex. Columnar organization and organization according to depth. *J. Neurophysiol.* **33**: 172–187.

Allison, A.C. (1953) The morphology of the olfactory system in the vertebrates. *Biol. Rev.* **28**: 195–244.

Balice-Gordon, R.J. and Lichtman, J.W. (1990) *In vivo* visualization of the growth of pre- and postsynaptic elements of neuromuscular junctions in the mouse. *J. Neurosci.* **10**: 894–908.

Balice-Gordon, R.J. and Lichtman, J.W. (1993) *In vivo* observations of pre- and postsynaptic changes during the transition from multiple to single innervation at developing neuromuscular junctions. *J. Neurosci.* **13**: 834–855.

Barde, Y.-A. (1989) Trophic factors and neuronal survival. *Nature* **2**: 1525–1534.

Barlow, H.B. (1975) Visual experience and cortical development. *Nature* **258**: 199–204.

Bartfeld, E. and Grinvald, A. (1992) Relationshps between orientation-preference pinwheels, cytochrome oxidase blobs, and ocular dominance columns in primate striate cortex. *Proc. Natl. Acad. Sci.* **89**: 11905–11909.

Belford, G.R. and Killackey, H.P. (1979) The development of vibrissae representation in subcortical trigeminal centers of the neonatal rat. *J. Comp. Neurol.* **188**: 63–74.

Benoit, P. and Changeux, J.-P. (1975) Consequences of tenotomy on the evolution of multi-innervation at the regenerating neuromuscular junction of the rat. *Brain Res.* **149**: 89–96.

Blasdel, C.G. and Salama, G. (1986) Voltage-sensitive dyes reveal a modular organization in monkey striate cortex. *Nature (Lond)* **32**: 579–585.

Bliss, T.V.P. and Collinridge, G.L. (1993) A synaptic model of memory: long-term potentiation in the hippocampus. *Nature* **361**: 31–39.

Brown, M.C. (1984) Sprouting of motor nerves in adult muscles: A recapitulation of ontogeny. *Trends in Neurosci.* **7**: 10–14.

Brown, M.C., Holland, R.L. and Hopkins, W.G. (1981) Motor nerve sprouting. *Ann. Rev. Neurosci.* **4**: 17–42.

Brown, M.C. and Ironton, R. (1977) Motor neurone sprouting induced by prolonged tetrodotoxin block of nerve action potentials. *Nature* **265**: 459–461.

Brown, M.C., Jansen, J.K.S. and Van Essen, D.C. (1976) Polyneuronal innervation of skeletal muscle in new-born rats and its elimination during maturation. *J. Physiol. (Lond)* **261**: 387–422.

Burke, R.E. (1983) Motor units: anatomy, physiology, and functional organization. In: *Handbook of Physiology – The Nervous System II*, Chapter 10, pp. 345–422. Bethesda: American Physiological Society.

Caldwell, J.H. and Ridge, R.M.A.P. (1983) The effects of deafferentation and spinal cord transection on synapse elimination in developing rat muscles. *J. Physiol. (Lond)* **339**: 145–159.

Changeux, J.-P. (1985) *Neuronal Man: The Biology of Mind*. Transl. by L. Garey. New York: Pantheon.

Changeux, J.-P., Courrège, P. and Danchin, A. (1973) A theory of the epigenesis of neuronal networks by selective stabilization of synapses. *Proc. Natl. Acad. Sci.* **70**: 2974–2978.

Changeux, J.-P. and Danchin, A. (1976) Selective stabilisation of developing synapses as a mechanism for the specification of neuronal networks. *Nature* **264**: 705–712.

Close, R.L. (1972) Dynamic properties of mammalian skeletal muscles. *Physiol. Rev.* **52**: 129–197.

Conel, J.L. (1939–1967) *The Postnatal Development of the Human Cerebral Cortex*, Volumes 1–8. Cambridge, MA: Harvard University Press.

Corsi, P. (1991) *The Enchanted Loom: Chapters in the History of Neuroscience* (Corsi, P., Ed.). New York: Oxford University Press.

Cott, H.B. and Huxley, J.S. (1940) *Adaptive Coloration in Animals*. London: Methuen.

Courtney, K. and Roper, S. (1976) Sprouting of synapses after partial denervation of frog cardiac ganglion. *Nature* **259**: 317–319.

Cowan, W.M. (1979) The development of the brain. *Sci. Amer.* **241**: 106–117.

Cragg, B.G. (1975) The development of synapses in the visual system of the cat. *J. Comp. Neurol.* **160**: 147–166.

Dawson, D.R. and Killackey, H.P. (1987) The organization and mutability of the forepaw and hindpaw representations in the somatosensory cortex of neonatal rat. *J. Comp. Neurol.* **256**: 246–256.

Dekaban, A.S. and Sadowsky, D. (1978) Changes in brain weights during the span of human life: relation of brain weight to body heights and body weights. *Ann. Neurol.* **4**: 345–356.

Donoghue, M.J., Morris-Valero, R., Johnson, Y.R., Merlie, J.P. and Sanes, J.R. (1992) Mammalian muscle cells bear a cell-autonomous, heritable memory of their rostrocaudal position. *Cell* **69**: 67–77.

Dunn, J. and Plomin, R. (1990) *Separate Lives*. New York: Basic Books.

Edelman, G.M. (1978) Group selection and phasic reentrant signalling: a theory of higher brain function. In: *The Mindful Brain: Cortical Organization and the Group-Selective Theory of Higher Brain Function* (Edelman, G.M. and Mountcastle, V.B., Eds.), pp. 55–100. Cambridge, MA: MIT Press.

Edelman, G.M. (1987) *Neural Darwinism: The Theory of Neuronal Group Selection*. New York: Basic Books.

Forehand, C.J. (1985) Density of somatic innervation on mammalian autonomic ganglion cells is inversely related to dendritic complexity and preganglionic convergence. *J. Neurosci.* **5**: 3403–3408.

Forehand, C.J. (1987) Ultrastructural analysis of the distribution of synaptic boutons from labeled preganglionic axons on rabbit ciliary neurons. *J. Neurosci.* **7**: 3274–3281.

Forehand, C.J. and Purves, D. (1984) Regional innervation of rabbit ciliary ganglion cells by the terminals of preganglionic axons. *J. Neurosci.* **4**: 1–12.

Furuno, K. Goodman, M.N. and Goldberg, A.L. (1990) Role of different proteolytic systems in the degradation of muscle proteins during denervation atrophy. *J. Biol. Chem.* **265**: 8550–8557.

Gazzaniga, M.S. (1993) *Nature's Mind: The Biological Roots of Thinking, Emotions, Sexuality, Language, and Intelligence.* New York: Basic Books.

Goldberg, A.L., Etlinger, J.D., Goldspink, D.F. and Jablecki, C. (1975) Mechanism of work-induced hypertrophy of skeletal muscle. *Medicine and Science in Sports* **7**: 185–198.

Goldman, P.S. and Nauta, W.J.H. (1977) Columnar distribution of cortico-cortical fibres in the frontal association, limbic and motor cortex of the developing rhesus monkey. *Brain Res.* **122**: 393–413.

Goldman-Rakic, P.S. and Schwartz, M.L. (1982) Interdigitation of contralateral and ipsilateral columnar projections to frontal association cortex in primates. *Science* **216**: 755–757.

Golgi, C. (1874) Sulla fina struttura dei bulbi olfattorii. *Riv. Sper. Freniat. Med. leg Alien Ment.* **1**: 405–425.

Gould, S.J. (1977) *Ontogeny and Phylogeny.* Cambridge, MA: Harvard University Press.

Graybiel, A.M. and Ragsdale, Jr C.W. (1978) Histochemically distinct compartments in the striatum of human, monkey, and cat demonstrated by acetylthiocholinesterase staining. *Proc. Natl. Acad. Sci. USA.* **75**: 5723–5726.

Guillery, R.W. (1973) Binocular competition in the control of geniculate cell growth. *J. Comp. Neurol.* **144**: 117–130.

Gutierrez, G. Riddle, D.R. and Purves, D. (1993) Neural activity after nominal deprivation of the somatic sensory cortex: 3H 2-deoxyglucose evaluation in the rat. *Soc. Neurosci. Abstr.* **19**: 1569.

Hamburger, V. (1977) The developmental history of the motor neuron. The F.O. Schmitt Lecture in Neuroscience, 1976. *Neurosci. Res. Program Bull. 15 (Suppl. 3)*: 1–37.

Hebb, D.O. (1949) *The Organization of Behavior.* New York: Wiley.

Hendrickson, A.E. (1985) Dots, stripes and columns in monkey visual cortex. *Trends in Neurosci.* **7**: 406.

Hevner, R.F. and Wong-Riley, M.T.T. (1992) Entorhinal cortex of the human, monkey, and rat: Metabolic map as revealed by cytochrome oxidase. *J. Comp. Neurol.* **326**: 451–469.

Holland, R.L. and Brown, M.C. (1980) Postsynaptic transmission block can cause terminal sprouting of a motor nerve. *Science* **207**: 649–651.

Horton, J.C. (1984) Cytochrome oxidase patches: A new cytoarchitectonic feature of monkey visual cortex. *Phil. Trans. R. Soc.
Lond. B* **304**: 199–253.

Hubel, D.H. (1982) Exploration of the primary visual cortex, 1955–
78. *Nature* **299**: 515–524.

Hubel, D.H. (1988) *Eye, Brain, and Vision.* Scientific American
Library Series. New York: W.H. Freeman.

Hubel, D.H. and Wiesel, T.N. (1962) Receptive fields, binocular
interaction and functional architecture in the cat's visual cortex. *J.
Physiol.* **160**: 106–154.

Hubel, D.H. and Wiesel, T.N. (1963) Receptive fields of cells in
striate cortex of very young, visually inexperienced kittens. *J.
Neurophysiol.* **26**: 994–1002.

Hubel, D.H. and Wiesel, T.N. (1963) Shape and arrangement of
columns in cat's striate cortex. *J. Physiol.* **165**: 559–568.

Hubel, D.H. and Wiesel, T.N. (1965) Binocular interaction in striate
cortex of kittens reared with artificial squint. *J. Neurophysiol.* **28**:
1041–1059.

Hubel, D.H. and Wiesel, T.N. (1977) Functional architecture of
macaque monkey cortex. *Proc. R. Soy. Lond. B* **198**: 1–59.

Hubel, D.H., Wiesel, T.N. and LeVay, S. (1977) Plasticity of ocular
dominance columns in the monkey striate cortex. *Phil. Trans. R.
Soc. Lond. B.* **278**: 377–409.

Hume, R.I. and Purves, D. (1981) Geometry of neonatal neurones
and the regulation of synapse elimination. *Nature* **293**: 469–471.

Hume, R.I. and Purves, D. (1983) Apportionment of the terminals
from single preganglionic axons to target neurones in the rabbit
ciliary ganglion. *J. Physiol.* **338**: 259–275.

Imig, T.J. and Adrián, I. (1977) Binaural columns in the primary
field (A1) of cat auditory cortex. *Brain Res.* 138: 241–257.

Imig, T.J. and Brugge, J.F. (1978) Sources and terminations of
callosal axons related to binaural and frequency maps in primary
auditory cortex of the cat. *J. Comp. Neurol.* **182**: 637–660.

Jackson, P.C. (1983) Reduced activity during development delays in
normal rearrangement of synapses in the rabbit ciliary ganglion.
J. Physiol. (Lond) **345**: 319–327.

Johnson, D.A. and Purves, D. (1981) Post-natal reduction of neural
unit size in the rabbit ciliary ganglion. *J. Physiol.* **318**: 143–159.

Johnson, Jr, E.M., Chang, J.Y., Koike, T. and Martin, D.P. (1989)

Why do neurons die when deprived of trophic factor. *Neurobiol. of Aging* **10**: 549–552.

Johnson, J.S. and Newport, E.L. (1989) Critical period effects in second language learning: The influence of maturational state on the acquisition of English as a second language. *Cog. Psychol.* **21**: 60–99.

Jones, D.A., Rutherford, D.M. and Parker, D.F. (1989) Physiological changes in skeletal muscle as a result of strength training. *Quart. J. Exp. Physiol.* **74**: 233–256.

Jones, E.G., Burton, H. and Porter, R. (1975) Commissural and cortico-cortical 'columns' in the somatic sensory cortex of primates. *Science* **100**: 572–574.

Juraska, J.M. (1987) The structure of the rat cerebral cortex: Effects of gender and the environment. In: *The Cerebral Cortex of the Rat* (Kolb, B. and Tees, R.C., Eds.), pp. 484–505. Cambridge, MA: MIT Press.

Kaprielian, Z. and Patterson, P.H. (1993) Surface and cytoskeletal markers of rostrocaudal position in the mammalian nervous system. *J. Neurosci.* **13**: 2495–2508.

Krogman, W.M. (1941) Tabulae Biologicae. In: *Growth of Man* (Denzer, H., Koningsberger, V.J. and Vonk, H.J., Eds.), Vol. XX. Den Haag.

LaMantia, A.-S., Pomeroy, S. and Purves, D. (1992) Vital imaging of glomeruli in the mouse olfactory bulb. *J. Neurosci.* **12**: 976–988.

LaMantia, A.-S. and Purves, D. (1989) Development of glomerular pattern visualized in the olfactory bulbs of living mice. *Nature* **341**: 646–649.

Langley, J.N. (1895) Note on regeneration of pre-ganglionic fibres of the sympathetic. *J. Physiol. (Lond)* **18**: 280–284.

Langley, J.N. (1897) On the regeneration of pre-ganglionic and post-ganglionic visceral nerve fibres. *J. Physiol. (Lond)* **22**: 215–230.

LeVay, S., Stryker, M.P. and Shatz, C.J. (1978) Ocular dominance columns and their development in layer V of the cat's visual cortex: a quantitative study. *J. Comp. Neurol.* **179**: 223–244.

Levi-Montalcini, R. (1987) The nerve growth factor: Thirty-five years later. *EMBO J.* **6**: 1145–1154.

Lichtman, J.W. (1977) The reorganization of synaptic connexions in the rat submandibular ganglion during postnatal development. *J. Physiol. (Lond)* **273**: 155–177.

Lichtman, J.W. (1980) On the predominantly single innervation of submandibular ganglion cells in the rat. *J. Physiol. (Lond)* **302**: 121–130.

Lichtman, J.W. and Purves, D. (1983) Activity-mediated neural change. *Nature* **301**: 563–564.

Livingstone, M.S. and Hubel, D.H. (1984) Anatomy and physiology of a color system in the primate visual cortex. *J. Neurosci.* **4**: 309–356.

Livingstone, M.S. and Hubel, D.H. (1987) Connections between layer 4B of area 17 and the thick cytochrome oxidase strips of area 18 in the squirrel monkey. *J. Neurosci.* **7**: 3371–3377.

Lorente de Nó, R. (1922) La corteza cerebral del ratón. *Trab. Lab. Invest. Biol. (Madr)* **20**: 41–78.

Lorente de Nó, R. (1949) The structure of cerebral cortex. In: *Physiology of the Nervous System*, 3rd Edition (Fulton, J. Ed.), pp. 288–330. New York: Oxford University Press.

Loughlin, S.E. and Fallon, J.H. (Eds.) (1993) *Neurotrophic Factors*. San Diego, CA: Academic Press, Harcourt Brace Jovanovich.

Madison, D.V., Malenka, R.C. and Nicoll, R.A. (1991) Mechanisms underlying long-term potentiation of synaptic transmission. *Ann. Rev. Neurosci.* **14**: 329–397.

Maffei, L., Berardi, N., Domenici, L., Parisi, V. and Pizzorusso, T. (1992) Nerve growth factor (NGF) prevents the shift in ocular dominance distribution of visual cortical neurons in monocularly deprived rats. *J. Neurosci.* **12**: 4651–4662.

Mata, M., Fink, D.J., Gainer, H., Smith, C.B., Davidsen, L., Savaki, H., Scwarts, W.J. and Sokoloff, L. (1980) Activity-dependent energy metabolism in rat posterior pituitary primarily reflects sodium pump activity. *J. Neurochem.* **24**: 213–215.

Megirian, D., Weller, L., Martin, G.F. and Watson, C.R.R. (1977) Aspects of laterality in the marsupial *Trichosurus vulpecula* (brush-tailed possum). *Ann. NY Acad. Sci.* **299**: 197–212.

Meisami, E. and Sendera, T.J. (1993) Morphometry of rat olfactory bulbs stained by cytochrome oxidase reveals that the entire population of glomeruli forms early in the neonatal period. *Dev. Brain Res.* **71**: 253–257.

Mountcastle, V.B. (1957) Modality and topographic properties of single neurons of cat's somatic sensory cortex. *J. Neurophysiol.* **20**: 408–434.

Murphy, K.M., Van Sluyters, R.C. and Jones, D.G. (1990) Cytochrome-oxidase activity in cat visual cortes: Is it periodic? *Soc. Neurosci. Abstr.* **16** (part 1): 292.

Njå, A. and Purves, D. (1978) The effects of nerve growth factor and its antiserum on synapses in the superior cervical ganglion of the guinea pig. *J. Physiol.* **277**: 53–75.

O'Brien, R.A.D., Ostberg, A.J.C. and Vrbová, G. (1978) Observations on the elimination of polyneural innervation in developing mammalian skeletal muscle. *J. Physiol.* **282**: 571–582.

Olson, L. and Malmfors, T. (1970) Growth characteristics of adrenergic nerves in the adult rat. Fluorescence, histochemical, and ^{3}H–noradrenaline uptake studies using tissue transplantations to the anterior chamber of the eye. *Acta Physiol. Scand., Suppl.* **348**: 1–111.

Pakkenberg, H. and Voigt, J. (1964) Brain weight of the Danes. *Acta. Anat.* **56**: 297–307.

Penfield, W. and Boldrey, E. (1937) Somatic motor and sensory representation in the cerebral cortex of man as studied by electrical stimulation. *Brain* **60**: 389–443.

Pomeroy, S.L., LaMantia, A.-S. and Purves, D. (1990) Postnatal construction of neural circuitry in the mouse olfactory bulb. *J. Neurosci.* **10**: 1952–1966.

Purves, D. (1975) Functional and structural changes in mammalian sympathetic neurones following interruption of their axons. *J. Physiol.* **252**: 405–426.

Purves, D. (1977) The formation and maintenance of synaptic connections. In: *The Function and Formation of Neural Systems* (Stent, G.S., Ed.), pp. 21–49. Berlin: Dahlem Konferenzen.

Purves, D. (1983) Modulation of neuronal competition by postsynaptic geometry in autonomic ganglia. *Trends in Neurosci.* **6**: 10–16.

Purves, D. (1986) The trophic theory of neural connections. *Trends in Neurosci.* **9**: 486–489.

Purves, D. (1988) *Body and Brain: A Trophic Theory of Neural Connections.* Harvard University Press.

Purves, D., Hadley, R.D. and Voyvodic, J.T. (1986) Dynamic changes in the dendritic geometry of individual neurons visualized over periods of up to three months in the superior cervical ganglion of living mice. *J. Neurosci.* **6**: 1051–1060.

Purves, D. and Hume, R.I. (1981) The relation of postsynaptic geometry to the number of presynaptic axons that innervate autonomic ganglion cells. *J. Neurosci.* **1**: 441–452.

Purves, D. and LaMantia, A.-S. (1993) The development of blobs in the monkey visual cortex. *J. Comp. Neurol.* **334**: 169–175.

Purves, D. and Lichtman, J.W. (1980) Elimination of synaptic connections in the developing nervous system. *Science* **210**: 153–157.

Purves, D. and Lichtman, J.W. (1985a) *Principles of Neural Development.* Sunderland, MA: Sinauer Associates.

Purves, D. and Lichtman, J.W. (1985b) Geometrical differences among homologous neurons in mammals. *Science* **228**: 298–302.

Purves, D., Riddle, D. and LaMantia, A.-S. (1992) Iterated patterns of brain circuitry (or how the cortex gets its spots). *Trends in Neurosci.* **15**: 362–368.

Purves, D., Riddle, D.R.R., White, L.W., Gutierrez, G. and LaMantia, A.-S. (in press) Categories of cortical structure. *Prog. in Brain Res.*

Purves, D., Rubin, E., Snider, W.D. and Lichtman, J.W. (1986) Relation of animal size to convergence, divergence and neuronal number in peripheral sympathetic pathways. *J. Neurosci.* **6**: 158–163.

Purves, D. and Sanes, J.R. (1987) The 1986 Nobel Prize in Physiology or Medicine. *Trends in Neurosci.* **10**: 231–235.

Purves, D. Snider, W.D. and Voyvodic, J.T. (1988) Trophic regulation of nerve cell morphology and innervation in the autonomic nervous system. *Nature* **336**: 123–128.

Purves, D. and Voyvodic, J. (1987) Imaging mammalian nerve cells and their connections over time in living animals. *Trends in Neurosci.* **10**: 398–404.

Purves, D., Voyvodic, J.T., Magrassi. L. and Yawo, H. (1987) Nerve terminal re-modeling visualized in living mice by repeated examination of the same neuron. *Science* **238**: 1122–1126.

Raichle, M.E. (1986) Neuroimaging. *Trends in Neurosci.* **9**: 525.

Rakic, P. (1974) Neurons in rhesus monkey visual cortex: Systematic relation between time of origin and eventual disposition. *Science* **183**: 425–427.

Rakic, P. (1985) Limits of neurogenesis in primates. *Science* **227**: 1054–1056.

Ramon-Moliner, E. (1972) Acetylthiocholinesterase distribution in the brain stem of the cat. *Anat. EntwGesh.* **46**: 1–53.

Redfern, P.A. (1970) Neuromuscular transmission in new-born rats. *J. Physiol. (Lond)* **209**: 701–709.

Riddle, D.R., Gutierrez, G., Zheng, D., White, L., Richards, A. and Purves, D. (1993) Differential metabolic and electrical activity in the somatic sensory cortex of the developing rat. *J. Neurosci.* **13**: 4193–4213.

Riddle, D., Richards, A., Zsuppan, F. and Purves, D. (1992) Growth of the rat somatic sensory cortex and its constituent parts during postnatal development. *J. Neurosci.* **12**: 3509–3524.

Roper, S. and Ko, C.-P. (1978) Synaptic remodeling in the partially denervated parasympathetic ganglion in the heart of the frog. In: *Neuronal Plasticity* (Cotman, C.W., Ed.), pp. 1–25. New York: Raven Press.

Sherman, S.M. and Spear, P.D. (1983) Organization of visual pathways in normal and visually deprived cats. *Physiol. Rev.* **62**: 738–854.

Snider, W.D. (1988) Nerve growth factor promotes dendritic arborization of sympathetic ganglion cells in developing mammals. *J. Neurosci.* **8**: 2628–2634.

Sokoloff, L. (1977) Relation between physiological function and energy metabolism in the central nervous syustem. *J. Neurochem.* **29**: 13–26.

Sokoloff, L. (1978) *Metabolic Probes of Central Nervous System Activity in Experimental Animals and Man.* Sunderland, MA: Sinauer Associates.

Sokoloff, L. (1979) Mapping of local cerebral functional activity by measurement of local cerebral glucose utilization with (^{14}C) deoxyglucose. *Brain* **102**: 653–668.

Sokoloff, L. (1981) Localization of functional activity in the central nervous system by measurement of glucose utilization with radioactive deoxyglucose. *J. Cereb. Blood Flow Metab.* **1**: 7–36.

Sperry, R.W. (1963) Chemoaffinity in the orderly growth of nerve fiber patterns and connections. *Proc. Natl. Acad. Sci.* **50**: 703–710.

Stevens, P.S. (1974) *Patterns in Nature.* Boston, MA: Little, Brown and Company.

Suzue, T., Kaprielian, Z. and Patterson, P.H. (1990) A monoclonal antibody that defines rostrocaudal gradients in the mammalian nervous system. *Neuron* **5**: 421–431.

Tees, R.C. (1990) Experience, perceptual competence, and rat cortex. In: *The Cerebral Cortex of the Rat* (Kolb, B. and Tees, R.C., Eds.), pp. 507–536. Cambridge, MA: MIT Press.

Thoenen, H. (1991) The changing scene of neurotrophic factors. *Trends in Neurosci.* **14**: 165–170.

Thompson, W.J. (1983) Synapse elimination in neonatal rat muscle is sensitive to pattern of muscle use. *Nature* **302**: 614–616.

Thompson, W.J., Kuffler, D.P. and Jansen, J.K.S. (1979) The effect of prolonged, reversible block of nerve impulses on the elimination of polyneural innervation of new-born rat skeletal muscle fibers. *Neurosci.* **4**: 271–281.

Tinbergen, N. (1969) *Curious Naturalists.* Garden City, NY: Doubleday.

Tower, S.S. (1939) The reaction of muscle to denervation. *Physiol. Rev.* **19**: 1–48.

Vincent, S.B. (1912) The function of the vibrissae in the behavior of the white rat. *Behav. Monogr.* **1**: 1–18.

Voyvodic, J.T. (1987) Development and regulation of dendrites in the rat superior cervical ganglion. *J. Neurosci.* **7**: 904–912.

Voyvodic, J.T. (1989) Peripheral target regulation of dendritic geometry in the rat superior cervical ganglion. *J. Neurosci.* **9**: 1997–2010.

Wallace, M.N. (1987) Histochemical demonstration of sensory maps in the rat and mouse cerebral cortex. *Brain Res.* **418**: 178–182.

Weibel, E.R. (1984) *The Pathway for Oxygen: Structure and Function in the Mammalian Respiratory System.* Cambridge, MA: Harvard University Press.

Welker, C. (1971) Microelectrode delineation of fine grain somatotopic organization of SmI cerebral neocortex in albino rat. *Brain Res.* **26**: 259–275.

Wiesel, T.N. (1982) Postnatal development of the visual cortex and the influence of environment. *Nature* **299**: 583–591.

Wiesel, T.N. and Hubel, D.H. (1963) Single cell responses in striate cortex of kittens deprived of vision in one eye. *J. Neurophysiol.* **26**: 1003–1017.

Wong-Riley, M.T.T. (1989) Cytochrome oxidase: An endogenous metabolic marker for neuronal activity. *Trends in Neurosci.* **12**: 94–101.

Wong-Riley, M.T.T., Tripathi, S.C., Trusk, T.C. and Hoppe, D.A. (1989) Effect of retinal impulse blockage on cytochrome oxidase-rich zones in the macaque striate cortex: I. Quantitative electron-microscopic (EM) analysis of neurons. *Visual Neurosci.* **2**: 483–497.

Woolsey, C.N. (1958) Organization of somatic sensory and motor areas of the cerebral cortex. In: *Biological and Biochemical Bases of Behavior* (Harlow, H.F. and Woolsey, C.N., Eds.), pp. 63–82. Madison, WI: University of Wisconsin Press.

Woolsey, T.A. and Van der Loos, H. (1970) The structural organization of layer IV in the somatosensory region (S1) of mouse cerebral cortex. *Brain Res.* **17**: 205–242.

Woolsey, T.A., Welker, C. and Schwartz, R.H. (1975) Comparative anatomical studies of the SmI face cortex with special reference to the occurrence of 'barrels' in layer IV. *J. Comp. Neurol.* **164**: 79–94.

Yawo, H. (1987) Changes in the dendritic geometry of mouse superior cervical ganglion cells following postganglionic axotomy. *J. Neurosci.* **7**: 3703–3711.

Young, J.Z. (1973) Memory as a selective process. In: *Australian Academy of Science Report: Symposium on Biological Memory*, pp. 25–45. Canberra: Australian Academy of Science.

Young, J.Z. (1979) Learning as a process of selection and amplification. *J. Roy. Soc. Med.* **72**: 801–814.

Zheng, D., LaMantia, A.-S. and Purves, D. (1991) Specialized vascularization of the primate visual cortex. *J. Neurosci.* **11**: 2622–2629.

Index